PENGUIN BOOKS

THE TRUE HISTORY OF THE ELEPHANT MAN

Michael Howell, who lived at Dudley in the West Midlands, was educated at Dudley Grammar School before he went on to study medicine at the University of Birmingham. He qualified in 1954 and then, during the course of his national service, became medical officer in the 2nd Battalion Grenadier Guards. After specializing in children's diseases for a time, he made the decision in 1960 to go into general practice, in which he continued until his death in 1986.

Peter Ford, who lives at Sudbury in Suffolk, served as a national serviceman in the Royal Artillery in Malaya. He then worked in publishing as an editor for twelve years before becoming a freelance writer and editor, specializing in editorial consultancy and co-authorship. He has written for collectors and has a particular interest in the history of popular entertainment. He wrote, with Max Wall, *The Fool on the Hill*, the autobiography of the great comedian, and, more recently, *Rings and Curtains: Family and Personal Memoirs*, with the veteran acrobat and actor, Jack Le White.

Michael Howell began his research into the life of Joseph Merrick, the Elephant Man, with the idea of writing an article. His findings eventually led to his collaboration with Peter Ford. They also worked together on a recasting of Merrick's story for children and a collection of documentary medical detective stories called *Medical Mysteries* (retitled *The Ghost Disease* in its paperback edition).

The True History of the Elephant Man

New Edition, Extensively Revised with Much Fresh Information

MICHAEL HOWELL AND PETER FORD

PENGUIN BOOKS

PENGUIN BOOKS

Published by the Penguin Group
Penguin Books Ltd, 27 Wrights Lane, London w8 5tz, England
Penguin Books USA Inc., 375 Hudson Street, New York, New York 10014, USA
Penguin Books Australia Ltd, Ringwood, Victoria, Australia
Penguin Books Canada Ltd, 10 Alcorn Avenue, Toronto, Ontario, Canada m4v 3b2
Penguin Books (NZ) Ltd, 182–190 Wairau Road, Auckland 10, New Zealand

Penguin Books Ltd, Registered Offices: Harmondsworth, Middlesex, England

First published by Allison & Busby 1980
Published in Penguin Books 1980
Second (illustrated) edition published 1983
Published simultaneously by Allison & Busby
Third edition published 1992
1 3 5 7 9 10 8 6 4 2

Typeset by DatIX International Limited, Bungay, Suffolk
Filmset in 10/12 pt Monophoto Times
Printed in England by Clays Ltd, St Ives plc

For Greta, and in memory of Michael

Contents

List of Plates

Preface and Acknowledgements

The first edition of *The True History of the Elephant Man* was published in the spring of 1980. The previous autumn, while the book was in the press, Bernard Pomerance's play, *The Elephant Man* (until then known mainly from 'art theatre' productions), was presented on Broadway. There it met with considerable popular success and in due course a Tony award, besides giving David Bowie his first serious stage role when he took over the lead. In the summer of 1980, the play began a long-running production at the National Theatre in London, and that autumn David Lynch's film, *The Elephant Man*, was released. There were few evident connections in the backgrounds to these events. It seemed more to be a synchronizing of several lines of coincidence.

The extraordinary concentration of interest in the life of Joseph Carey Merrick that was caused by these treatments, imaginative and documentary, had two main effects. First, it established the story itself as an invariably moving myth in popular consciousness. Secondly, it led, directly and indirectly, to further details of Merrick's life emerging from obscurity, sometimes from unexpected sources.

So far as the facts in the case are concerned, Dr Howell and I had called our book a 'true' history. Even if that, too, carried a mythic resonance in the style, say, of the balladeers of earlier times, it was disconcerting to find how many of our assumptions and inferences came to need reappraisal and adjustment. We had striven to include in our account no statements beyond those that could be justified from documentary record. Yet interpretation may only proceed in line with the facts as known. A shifting pattern of facts, in any context, becomes a part of the process of understanding events.

As for the mythic dimension – and here it is essential not to fall into the common error of calling myth *per se* 'untrue' – it has resulted in the story of the Elephant Man acquiring a whole cultural history in its own right. It was a process that may be said to have begun in 1923 when Sir Frederick Treves's *The Elephant Man and Other Reminiscences* was published, and to have received a boost along the way in 1971 with the publication of Ashley Montagu's *The Elephant Man: A Study in Human Dignity*. Its manifestations have been remarkably varied.*

John Hinkley, for instance, the schizophrenic young man who in 1981 made an attempt with a firearm on the life of President Reagan, was found to have written poems that contained the cryptic thought: 'Perhaps the Elephant Man would understand my dilemma . . . it's all a matter of face to face communication.' A cycle of poems, *Words for Elephant Man*, was published in 1983 by the American poet, Kenneth Sherman. In 1988, Michael Cavalli, an amateur composer, spent his life savings on hiring an orchestra and the Central Hall, Westminster, to hear a performance of his *Symphonic Poem*, also based on the Elephant Man's life. The previous year the singer and performer, Michael Jackson, had been reported to have made the London Hospital an offer of $500,000, later expanded to $1,000,000, if they would sell him Merrick's skeleton.

This episode in particular provoked a good deal of ill-informed speculation in the British press for a day or two. It has subsequently been claimed that Jackson's bids were no more than a publicity stunt. Nevertheless his visits to view the skeleton, and his obsession, seem to have been real enough. Yet if the episode was nothing more than a prank to do with image making, then clearly it misfired. The impression created was of a bizarre spectacle, as if a demonic emissary were attempting, almost a century on, to reclaim Merrick's bones for show business.

The untimely death of Michael Howell in 1986 deprived me of a

---

* Those who may wish to read more deeply into the mythologizing elements (both purposeful and involuntary) involved in versions of and responses to Merrick's story, will find a wealth of material usefully summarized and analysed in Peter W. Graham's and Fritz H. Oehlschlaeger's recent study, *Articulating the Elephant Man: Joseph Merrick and His Interpreters*.

friend and colleague, and of many continuing opportunities for entertaining and wondering discussion. We did, of course, work together on the revised text for the 1983 edition, but its print numbers were relatively restricted and it was the original 1980 trade edition that continued to be most widely available during the rest of the decade. In preparing what is therefore the third edition for publication, I have been conscious of the absence of Michael's shrewd asides and wise counsel, though I hope he would have approved of the result. It chronicles and attempts to balance all the facts in Merrick's life as they are presently known. Since it was Michael Howell who, some time in the late 1960s, set out on the trail of the Elephant Man during his precious afternoons off from a demanding Black Country practice, I feel it appropriate that it should be dedicated both to his widow and his own memory.

Considering the wealth of fresh information that came to the surface during the 1980s, it would perhaps be rash to speculate that we now know most of what we are ever likely to know of Joseph Merrick in a documentary sense. On the other hand, it is clear that the history of his story is far from over and may, indeed, remain open-ended indefinitely. In certain of its aspects, it seems firmly set in the Victorian matrix of its origins, for even the elements of fairy tale and melodrama are naturally there in the known details and have no need of embroidering. In other aspects, its time-transcending qualities possess an influence to teach, to change attitudes towards the disabled and malformed, perhaps even to help to heal the psychic traumas that must always be a hidden component in physical disability. During fifteen years of living with Joseph Merrick's story, and never ceasing to be moved by it, I have inevitably had my fanciful moments of feeling that is what he would wish.

This book has evolved into its present state through three editions; its list of acknowledgements is therefore long. The quotation from the journal kept by Lady Geraldine Somerset for the Duchess of Cambridge is reproduced by gracious permission of Her Majesty the Queen. It was Georgina Battiscombe, the biographer of Queen Alexandra, who drew attention to this in the Royal Archives, Windsor Castle Library, and Sir Robin Mackworth-Young, the then librarian, supplied a copy of the text.

The London Hospital kindly gave permission to quote from the Minutes of the London Hospital House Committee. Professor Gordon Seward, CBE, of the London Hospital Medical College, has continued to be unstinting in the way he has given encouragement and time in checking and offering criticisms of the text, both of the original draft and of the rewriting made necessary by developments in the hypothetical medical picture during the 1980s. J. P. Entract, former librarian of the London Hospital Medical College, was patient and more than helpful over a long period, as was Percy Nunn, the former assistant curator of the college museum. The latter's son, David Nunn, has, as his successor as assistant curator, happily continued this tradition and maintained contact in mutual exchanges of fresh information. Margaret Robertson took photographs in the London Hospital Medical College Museum, and Julia Short searched the hospital's photographic archives for items of possible relevance.

There are many others to whom a special debt is owed, for kindness in general and for guidance in the direction of much particular information. These include: W. J. Barlow; Mrs Nellie Batchelor, who was kind enough to recount all she could remember of her uncle Walter Steel's recollections of meeting Merrick; David Braithwaite; Dr K. T. Brown; Colonel Rixon Bucknell, who helped to clarify the likely train ferry routes from the Continent to Harwich in 1886; Richard Carr-Gomm; G. W. Essex; William Dooley (Benson Dulay), who passed on information about his uncle Sam Roper's fair as well as family anecdotes originally told by his father Bertram Dooley of the time when he travelled with Merrick on the fairground circuits, and who made family photographs available; Mrs Marion Duck, who corresponded about her and Tom Norman's Noakes forebears and origins; Colin Eaton, who generously shared his researches in the Northamptonshire Records Office, drawing attention to the existence there of Lady Louisa Knightley's diaries and acting as an initial contact with the families of Bertram Dooley and Walter Steel; Dr Ron Finch, who, by his painstaking photographic skills, made some excellent prints out of apparently unpromising archive material, work later supplemented by Denis Clark and by Les Curtis of Chilton Colour Laboratories, Sudbury; Desmond Flower; E. R. Frizelle; John Garratt; Robert Geary;

the Great Eastern Railway Society, for help with amplifying earlier research, and whose members, L. D. Brooks and J. Sweszkowski, located some rare picture material; Peter Honri; Mrs Leila Hoskins, who provided information about her aunt, Mrs Leila Maturin (née Leila Scot Skirving), and a copy of the pamphlet reproduced here as Appendix Two, and who presented the authors with the only known surviving example of Merrick's correspondence; Winston F. Hughes, who offered an eyewitness description of Merrick's specially built bed; Mrs Margaret Hunter, who sent details of the book inscribed by Merrick for his cousin; Pat Kingston, who, with the help of Janice Tipping, typed the successive drafts of the first edition and handled much of the correspondence in the early stages; Mrs Kenneth Lindy, daughter of Dr Tuckett, who spoke of her father (and of his disappointment at Treves's failure to record his role in his version of the story) provided prints of the Elephant Man that had been among his papers; the staff and facilities of the London Library; Michelle Merrick, whose interest in and diligent researches into the Merrick family history have uncovered further details of value; the descendants of Tom Norman, among whom Tom Norman Jnr originally made his father's unpublished memoirs available, while Arthur Van Norman helped to round out details of the later days of the Silver King's career and George Barnum Norman kindly presented a copy of the published edition of the memoirs, including his additions, which also threw some new light on the story (and additionally made it at last possible to reconstruct the most probable sequence of events in Merrick's travels with the showmen); Michael Pointon; Nicholas Reed, who kindly allowed access to Treves's autographed manuscript of 'The Elephant Man', which was then in his possession, and to a collection of Treves's correspondence; W. H. Steel; Dr C. E. Taylor, possessor of the chair that his grandfather, William Taylor, adapted for Merrick's use; Dr Kate Thompson, former archivist of the Leicester Museum, and the staff of the Leicester Museum and Library; the descendants of Sam Torr, and especially Mrs Harry Heatherley (Patricia Torr), Mrs Hilda Metcalfe and Roy Torr, who made their collections of cuttings and family memorabilia fully available; and Frederick Treves, great-nephew of Sir Frederick Treves, who gave help and showed interest from a very early stage of the search for the Elephant Man.

PREFACE AND ACKNOWLEDGEMENTS

Finally, I would like to record my gratitude to the island of South Walls off Hoy in the Orkneys for providing the peace and seclusion in which to work on much of the revision for this edition.

Suffolk and Orkney   P.F.
1989–92

CHAPTER I

'The Great Freak of Nature –
Half-a-Man and Half-an-Elephant'

When the Elephant Man appeared as if from nowhere in a shop premises in the Whitechapel Road in London towards the end of November 1884, he was still in the early days of his career as a professional freak. His real name, as his birth certificate bears witness, was Joseph Carey Merrick, and his manager at that time was Mr Tom Norman, a showman who specialized in the display of freaks and novelties. The shop hired for his exhibition was then numbered 123 Whitechapel Road. The building survives today as one in a terraced row of early nineteenth-century shops, though it has since been renumbered as 259. The adjoining premises to its east side carried until recently the pawnbroker's emblem of three iron balls high up on the wall. To the west side lay the shop of Mr Michael Geary, fruiterer and greengrocer.

Directly across the road from the row of shops, on the other side of the wide thoroughfare, stands the imposing entrance to the London Hospital. The present front in fact dates from improvements made in 1891. In the 1880s the hospital displayed a long and imposing classical façade, set well back behind railings and with porters' lodges at the main gates. The whole effect was designed to inspire confidence in the capabilities of medical science as well as a measure of appropriate awe among the inhabitants of the district. It was the outward and visible sign of authoritarian benevolence and charity in an area that had for many decades experienced an intimate connection with deprivation and poverty: one in which successive waves of penniless immigrants settled alongside the original communities of London's poor; those who, in the definition of the great Victorian pioneer in social investigation, Henry Mayhew, 'Will work, cannot work and will not work.'

In such a district therefore Joseph Merrick arrived to fall under Tom Norman's care, it being hoped that the Elephant Man's impact on London would be profitable for them both. Outside the premises, across the shop front, leaving only the doorway clear, the showman hung a large canvas sheet painted with the startling image of a man half-way through the process of turning into an elephant and announcing that the same was to be seen within for the entrance price of twopence. If the artistry was rough, and the colours garish to sophisticated taste, the poster evidently had the sensational effect intended. A young surgeon from the London Hospital, Mr Frederick Treves, who visited the freakshow, could recall the poster in every vivid detail when he came to write about it some forty years later:

> This very crude production depicted a frightful creature that could only have been possible in a nightmare. It was the figure of a man with the characteristics of an elephant. The transfiguration was not far advanced. There was still more of the man than of the beast. This fact – that it was still human – was the most repellent attribute of the creature. There was nothing about it of the pitiableness of the misshapened or the deformed, nothing of the grotesqueness of the freak, but merely the loathing insinuation of a man being changed into an animal. Some palm trees in the background of the picture suggested a jungle and might have led the imaginative to assume that it was in this wild that the perverted object had roamed.

Whatever it was which could possibly be causing poor Merrick to take on an approximation to an elephant, in displaying him as a freak Mr Norman was working in an ancient tradition the roots of which lay far back in the history of fairgrounds and circuses in England. London in particular had been noted for its insatiable appetite for monsters since at least the days of Elizabeth I. As Henry Morley stated in his *Memoirs of Bartholomew Fair*, it was not merely the common throng who sought out a formidable diet of signs and wonders and supported popular fashions in the grotesque. Everyone in society, up to the level of its crowned head, 'shared in the tastes ... for men who could dance without legs, dwarfs, giants, hermaphrodites, or scaly boys'. He goes on to comment, writing his book in the late 1850s:

> The taste still lingers among uncultivated people in the highest and lowest ranks of life, but in the reign of William and Mary, or Queen Anne, it was almost universal. Bartholomew Fair, with all the prodigies exhibited therein, was not as it now would be, an annual display of things hardly to be seen out of a fair, but was, as far as Monsters went, only a yearly concentration into one spot of the entertainments that at other times were scattered over town and country.

Bartholomew Fair was officially opened each year on 23 August, the eve of Saint Bartholomew, and continued for two weeks. While the revels lasted, many poor tradesmen in the Smithfield area were glad to hire out a part of their premises for the display of some prodigy of nature. Prime sites were those shops or workrooms close to taverns, such as the premises where a 'changeling child' might be viewed,

> next door to the *Black Raven* in West Smithfield . . . being a living Skeleton, taken by a *Venetian* Galley, from a *Turkish* Vessel in the *Archipelago*. This is a Fairy Child, supposed to be born of *Hungarian* Parents, but chang'd in the Nursing, Aged Nine Years and more; not exceeding a foot and a half high. The Legs, Thighs and Arms are so very small, that they scarce exceed the bigness of a Man's Thumb, and the face no bigger than the Palm of one's hand.

On another occasion, 'next door to the *Golden Hart in West-Smithfield*', there was to be seen 'the Admirable Work of Nature, a Woman having Three Breasts; and each of them affording Milk at one time, or differently, according as they are made use of'.

Advancing sharply up the social scale, the West End of London featured its permanent exhibition halls available for hire to show-men. When, in 1826, the bookseller and radical pamphleteer William Hone interviewed Claude Amboise Seurat, the 'Anatomie Vivant; or Living Skeleton!' for the edification of readers of his periodical *The Every-day Book*, he visited him at Pall Mall in a room known as the Chinese Saloon. When Barnum brought

General Tom Thumb to London in 1844, the curiosity aroused was so phenomenal that he was able to engage the Egyptian Hall in Piccadilly. These remarkable premises were built in 1812 by William Bullock to show his own vast and miscellaneous collection of curiosities, the nucleus for which he gathered together during his earlier years as a silversmith in Liverpool when he bought rarities from sailors arriving at the port from exotic quarters of the globe.

The Egyptian Hall started life with cultural and educational pretensions, containing 'upwards of Fifteen Thousand Natural and Foreign Curiosities, Antiquities and Productions of the Fine Arts'. While these aspirations were never quite lost sight of, the lease passed into the hands of others and the Egyptian Hall became the recognized showplace for every nine-days' wonder expected to excite lively interest. Matters reached such a pitch that *Punch*, in 1847, suggested the existence of an epidemic of a new disease termed 'Deformito-mania' and published a cartoon satirizing the placards decorating the Egyptian Hall's façade.

It is a long walk from the West End to Whitechapel; but appropriately enough the route from Smithfield may be retraced back along Cheapside, through the City of London and eventually along the Whitechapel Road – appropriately, since this was the main route into London from East Anglia and the Eastern Counties. It was the route taken by the drovers who once walked herds of cattle for sale at Smithfield market to keep the metropolis supplied with fresh meat. The Whitechapel Road is still part of the main thoroughfare into the City of London for traffic from the east, and its exceptional width is a legacy of its origins as a droving road. It is this width, in turn, that has made it a natural location for the street market traders' stalls that continue to do business there, if they no longer do so in the colourful profusion which must have set the scene during the late nineteenth century.

There was another young surgeon who stumbled across the Elephant Man in his original London exhibition even before Frederick Treves. John Bland-Sutton, from the Middlesex Hospital, was in later years to become a consulting surgeon to the Middlesex Hospital, President of the Royal College of Surgeons, and a baronet, besides making a long-term study of the phenomenon of Siamese twins. In 1884 he had only just attained his fellowship of

4

the Royal College of Surgeons. As he recorded in his collection of autobiographical reminiscences, *The Story of a Surgeon*, he was in the habit of wandering out through the East End of London as far as the Mile End Road to satisfy a mixture of professional interest and idle curiosity:

> ... especially on Saturday nights, to see dwarfs, giants, fat-women, and monstrosities at the freak shows. There was a freak-museum at a public-house – The Bell and Mackerel, near the London Hospital. It was on one of these visits in 1884 I saw 'on show' opposite the London Hospital a repulsive human being known as the Elephant Man. The poor fellow, John [*sic*] Merrick – was deformed in body, face, head and limbs. His skin, thick and pendulous, hung in folds and resembled the hide of an elephant – hence his show-name.

In another autobiography, *A Labrador Doctor*, Sir Wilfred Grenfell, whose early medical training was gained at the London Hospital, made the suggestion that it was some medical students from the hospital who first went to view the Elephant Man in the exhibition shop, then returned to describe him to their surgeon-lecturer in anatomy, Frederick Treves. In his memoirs, the showman himself, Mr Tom Norman, remembered how

> ... there were, every week-day morning and afternoon until about 3 p.m., a number of students with white coats and no hats passing in and out of the London Hospital opposite for the purpose of what I then presumed, for to obtain refreshments, fresh air, etc. After a few had, out of curiosity, visited the exhibition, the wonderful sight of Meyrick [*sic*] soon spread among them, and no doubt that was the reason of Sir Frederick's visit ...

It was in fact Frederick Treves's house surgeon who first told him about the Elephant Man. Dr Reginald Tuckett was then twenty-four years old and employed by the hospital in the most junior of its appointments. He had begun his medical studies as an articled pupil to his brother-in-law, a doctor in the Welsh border country. To qualify for admission to the Medical Register, however, he came to the London Hospital to complete his training. It was now a little more than a year since he qualified, and he was employed by the hospital as house physician, house surgeon and resident accoucheur. The burden of his responsibilities did not, even so, prevent his being enticed across the road by the showman's poster. The graphic account of the exhibit he carried back to the hospital was compelling enough to prompt Treves into making his own pilgrimage to the north side of the Whitechapel Road to view the Elephant Man for himself.

When he arrived outside the shop, Treves says, it was to find the exhibition temporarily closed. Questioning a small boy who was hanging about on the pavement, he learnt where the showman might be found and persuaded the lad to seek him out where he was refreshing himself in one of the local taverns. The showman proved unhesitating when it came to striking a bargain: he would open the exhibition for a private viewing on condition that a special entrance fee of one shilling was paid. The scene was set for Frederick Treves's first encounter with Joseph Merrick, the Elephant Man.

The classic account of that meeting is contained in the title piece to *The Elephant Man and Other Reminiscences*. It is reproduced in its full text as the third appendix of the present book (pages 181–200). Within a well-told anecdote, Treves presents a series of vivid images; it is a powerful and unforgettable literary achievement. It may be that it rests a little heavily on melodrama, yet it remains as highly readable as when it was written and fully deserves to be read. On the other hand, it raises incidental questions about the relationship between objective truth and the validity of literary creation and is not to be regarded uncritically in that respect.

Treves was certainly not starting out to write fiction when, towards the end of his life, he finally set down the tale of the Elephant Man for inclusion in what was to be his last published work. The essay, however, is marked by a strong romanticizing tendency. There are obvious errors: the London Hospital does not, for instance, stand in the Mile End Road as he states in the opening sentence. There are numerous indications of a memory becoming overlaid over the years with small embellishing details that add colour and effect to the story-telling. Above all there is the curious fact that in the one and only place where Treves gives Joseph

Merrick a Christian name he calls him John. The detail seems doubly curious in that a whole segment of Treves's life and career came to be intertwined with the destiny of Joseph Merrick, and as matters turned out it was hardly a superficial relationship.

Might it have been that the facial distortions that were a part of Merrick's condition, and which made comprehensible speech extremely difficult for him, meant that Treves misheard? Did Treves hear 'Joseph' as 'John' during an early conversation and ever afterwards think of him as and call him 'John'? Yet others heard and recorded his name correctly, and to put down the error to a simple lapse of memory on Treves's part is an unconvincing explanation. From the very beginning of their relationship, Treves was writing of Merrick as 'John' in his technical papers. Did Merrick himself prefer the name? Evidently not, for he called himself Joseph and signed himself Joseph in the two examples of his handwriting that survive. Whatever the reason for the misnomer applied to Merrick, it has had one long-term consequence: almost every reference to the Elephant Man subsequently printed has repeated the error because the authors could not believe that someone of Treves's standing might be wrong on such a basic detail.

There is also the question of the identity of the shop where Tom Norman set up his exhibition. It was, says Treves, 'a vacant greengrocer's which was to let'. He goes on to sketch in a number of scenic props:

> The shop was empty and grey with dust. Some old tins and a few shrivelled potatoes occupied a shelf and some vague vegetable refuse the window.

Tom Norman was stung into writing an emphatic letter to the showman's paper the *World's Fair* when he first heard about Treves's essay, among the details he wished to correct being the fact that Merrick 'was not exhibited in an empty greengrocer's shop'.

> That shop was next door to the one in which he was exhibited and kept by a man named Geary, an Irishman, in the Whitechapel Road. The shop on the other side of the one we were showing was . . . a pawnbroker's. The premises used for the exhibition of Meyrick [*sic*] had for several years previously

been a waxworks museum, owned by a man named Cotton. I came to London and rented it from him, and removed Meyrick thereto ...

According to the *London Directory* for 1886, prepared in 1885, the greengrocer's opposite to the London Hospital was indeed kept by a Mr Michael Geary. It appears that he took possession of his shop towards the end of 1884, for the directory prepared in that year lists the occupier as a Mr William Parry. And next door but one to the greengrocer's there was, sure enough, the pawnbroker's. The shop premises at 123 Whitechapel Road, now 259, sandwiched between the pawnshop and the fruiterer's, is recorded in the directories as a glass warehouse belonging to Albert and Eli Shepherd. In view of Tom Norman's precise statement and the corroborative evidence from the directories, it seems it was the front portion of this shop that was sub-let to Mr Cotton for use as a waxworks museum. A waxworks museum certainly flourished opposite to the London Hospital, for in September 1888, in the midst of the Whitechapel murders committed by 'Jack the Ripper', a correspondent called John Law was writing in the columns of the *Pall Mall Gazette*:

There is at present almost opposite the London Hospital a ghastly display of the unfortunate woman murdered ... An old man exhibits these things, and while he points them out you will be tightly wedged in between a number of boys and girls, while a smell of death rises into your nostrils, and you feel as if your throat was filled up with fungus.

It was therefore not the greengrocer's door but the one to No. 123 Whitechapel Road that Tom Norman in due course unlocked and opened. Nevertheless we may continue, for the moment, to take Frederick Treves's account at face value. It was difficult for the visitor, ushered into the dark interior, to pick out anything at first, for the light from the window was obstructed by the large canvas sheet bearing its message to the passers-by in the street. The atmosphere was decidedly cold and damp and there was a faint but peculiarly unpleasant odour hanging in the air. The main part of the shop was bare and disused, but towards the back a cord had been suspended across the room from one side to the other, and from this there hung down what might have been a large red tablecloth to form an improvised screen.

As soon as they were in the shop Tom Norman went across to the screen and drew it aside. There in the half-light beyond sat the figure of the Elephant Man, seemingly remarkably small in contrast to the impression of something gigantic created by the poster. He was hunched up on a stool and held a brown blanket drawn well up about himself to cover his head and shoulders. The movement of the curtain did not seem to disturb him, for he continued to sit motionless and to stare at the blue flame of a gas burner arranged to heat a large brick balanced on a tripod before him. This was the only source of heat and light in the room. The very stillness of the almost diminutive figure awoke in Treves the feeling, as he said, that here was the very 'embodiment of loneliness'.

At this moment, Treves states, the showman suddenly called out a sharp instruction to the figure: 'Stand up!' speaking 'harshly', 'as if to a dog'. The description implies a brutal insensitivity on the part of the Elephant Man's keeper, as might be expected from someone who was dealing with a creature supposedly half-human, half-beast – a kind of urban Caliban. And then, as if reluctantly, the Elephant Man stirred and rose awkwardly to his feet, letting the blanket slip to the ground as he turned to face his exclusive audience. As the covering fell the source of the peculiar odour that hung in the air inside the shop became apparent, for the sickening stench evidently had its origins in the startling condition of the subject's body and intensified at once.

Treves's medical career had from its beginning been associated with the London Hospital. He had arrived as a medical student in 1871, become assistant surgeon in 1879 and been appointed full surgeon in this very year of 1884. Although he was still only thirty-one, his experience of the appalling range of physical horrors and injuries likely to be admitted into a foundation that existed to minister to the ills of an area containing some of the worst slums of Europe must have been considerable. It would be reasonable to expect him to be shock-proof, his nose used to such smells as gangrene, his eyes accustomed to the terrible facial injuries that could result from a fight with broken bottles in any London pub on a Saturday night. From what he says it is nevertheless clear that he was shaken by his first glimpse of Joseph Merrick; perhaps also taken unawares by his revulsion at the sickening stench given off by Merrick's body. He summed up his initial reaction in a memorable phrase: that Merrick seemed to him 'the most disgusting specimen of humanity'. 'At no time,' wrote Treves, 'had I met with such a degraded or perverted version of a human being as this lone figure displayed.'

As Treves stared, the Elephant Man began to turn slowly about so that his visitor might view him from all angles. The movement re-awakened the surgeon's clinical instincts and he noticed how the unfortunate creature showed signs of having at some time in life suffered a disease of the left hip; it had left him lame so that he needed to lean on a stick. With the return of a habit of scientific detachment, Treves began to make precise observations. Where he had been expecting to see a figure both monstrous and large, the Elephant Man was of quite a slight build, perhaps only a little over five foot two inches in height. The upper part of his body was unclothed to the waist, the lower half was clad in a pair of threadbare trousers that seemed to have 'once belonged to some fat gentleman's dress suit'. The feet were also naked, and his lameness became obvious as he stood there, his body slightly tilted to the left, his back twisted and bent.

More than anything else, it was the head that created such an amazing impression. It did indeed seem huge beyond Treves's most imaginative expectations: a misshapen mass of bony lumps and cauliflower-like growths of skin. It had the circumference of a man's waist, and the forehead was disfigured by bosses of bony material that bulged forward in great mounds, giving it an appearance something resembling a cottage loaf laid on its side. The greater mound pressed down upon the right eyebrow so that the eye on that side of the face was almost hidden.

The lower half of the face was itself compressed and distorted by a swelling of the right cheek, where a pink mass of flesh protruded from the mouth, forcing back the lips into inverted folds. Here was evidently the origin of the 'trunk' the poster artist had so graphically portrayed, if with a certain artistic licence to enhance its resemblance to an elephant's anatomy. There were other bony masses present on the top and side of the skull, but in these areas it was the skin that dominated, the flesh being raised up into heavy cauliflower-textured growths which hung down at the sides and back of the head.

Merrick's body itself was in no way spared. Masses of similar pendulous growths of skin hung down from the chest and back. Elsewhere it looked as though the skin was covered with fine warts. The right arm was enormous in size and virtually shapeless, the right hand being 'large and clumsy – a fin or paddle rather than a hand ... The thumb had the appearance of a radish, while the fingers might have been thick tuberous roots.' It was impossible to imagine such a limb being of much use to its owner. By contrast the left arm and hand looked completely normal, even delicate and feminine in their refinement. The feet, so far as Treves could make out, were as shapeless and deformed as the gross right arm.

The showman seemed to Treves to be unable or unwilling to pass on more than the most rudimentary information about his charge: that he was English born, that he was twenty-one years old and that his name, Treves claimed he told him, was John Merrick. For his own part, Treves felt a frustrating bafflement at the malformations he found himself observing. He was quite unable to account for the condition, to pin on it any label of medical diagnosis or recall ever having come across anything remotely like it in professional experience or theoretical training.

Treves was at the age of thirty-one already a figure to be reckoned with in the medical world. In 1881 he had been invited by the Royal College of Surgeons to give the Erasmus Wilson Lectures, a series of six lecture-demonstrations on specimens from the college's museum to be delivered before an audience consisting of some of the most distinguished surgeons in the country. He added to this honour the winning of the college's Jacksonian Prize in 1883 for an original essay on intestinal surgery. In the same year he published *Surgical Applied Anatomy*, a textbook that lost no time in establishing itself as both a standard reference work and a medical best-seller. If he was disconcerted by his bewilderment before the sorely afflicted frame of Joseph Merrick, he must have been stimulated by the challenge it presented to his diagnostic abilities and to his natural instincts as a scientific investigator.

The explanation offered by Mr Norman to account for his protégé's deformities at least had the virtue of simplicity. All this came about, he explained, as the consequence of an unfortunate accident. While the Elephant Man's mother was carrying him during the last few months of her pregnancy, she was knocked over and badly frightened by an elephant from a travelling menagerie. The shock sustained conveyed itself to the unborn child with the result they saw before them. (Dr Bland-Sutton also remembered this story in connection with his visit to the freakshow.) As will be seen, Merrick himself clung to it, finding it to contain a powerful degree of comfort. The extreme rarity of his sensational disorder was no doubt to be accounted for by the scarcity of runaway elephants in rural England.

Frederick Treves's interest in the case was quite naturally not concerned with exploring it as medical folk-belief. Ignoring the vagaries of superstition, his instincts were to seek to establish scientific fact and, if appropriate, to write up an account of these apparently undescribed abnormalities for publication. His mind was quite made up that he would like to take Merrick back across the road so that he might examine him in detail at leisure in his room in the London Hospital's Medical College. Tom Norman again proved ready to agree, perceiving some publicity value in the idea. But at this point, wrote Treves, 'I became at once conscious of a difficulty.'

Considerable problems were invariably to be encountered in transporting this startling being from place to place. The problem remained even when the distance concerned was no more than the few hundred yards to the door of the Medical College, which lay along Turner Street, on the south-west side of the London Hospital's main complex of buildings. For the Elephant Man to appear on the streets without concealment was to invite the instant assembling of a crowd. In the open, out of his refuge, Merrick's footsteps were invariably dogged by ever-increasing excitement and clamour, his progress hampered by eager, curious, shocked or frankly incredulous bystanders. The Elephant Man's journeyings abroad were, it seemed, in the habit of degenerating into public disturbances.

There was a solution to hand – at least, a partial solution – and this, said Treves, took the form of a special set of outdoor clothes the

Elephant Man possessed that concealed him from head to toe. The whole outfit consisted of three garments. First there came a pair of huge bag-like slippers in which the feet and lower legs could be encased. Then there was the voluminous black cloak, and this practically touched the ground when draped about its owner's shoulders. Treves could only remember having seen such a garment once before, and then it had been at a theatre, when it was 'wrapped about the figure of a Venetian bravo'. He found it difficult to imagine how the Elephant Man came by such a garment, yet the most extraordinary item of clothing remained the hat. It was shaped somewhat like a conventional peaked cap, and was also black in colour. Its dimensions, however, were vast, since it needed to be large enough to fit the Elephant Man's head. From the edge of the wide peak a brownish flannel pelmet hung down to conceal the face, but in this a horizontal slit was cut so Merrick could see where he was walking.

The sight of the Elephant Man limping slowly along in his outdoor clothing – a slight, bent figure leaning heavily on a stick and engulfed in a huge black cloak, the whole ensemble topped off by the great head in its 'pillar-box' hat – could, Treves remarked, have been only a degree or so less alarming than the appearance of the man unclothed. It was decided in the end that Merrick would wear outdoor garments for his visit to the Medical School, but that Treves would hire a cab to carry him from door to door and return him afterwards in the same way.

There remained only the need to ensure the smooth reception of the Elephant Man at the college. So that he might identify himself to the porter and avoid embarrassing delays or misunderstandings, Treves handed Merrick his visiting card. With this gesture the first meeting was over between Frederick Treves, a young surgeon whose ever more ambitious career was opening before him, and Joseph Merrick, the Elephant Man, a humble freak whose hopes for the future were altogether more modest in character.

CHAPTER 2

On the Threshold of Eminence

By any standards Treves cut an impressive figure. He might almost have posed for a monument to what it was possible to achieve by a combination of a peculiarly Victorian trio of virtues: industry, tenacity and talent. He had reached the age of thirty-one with his life a success story.

Treves was a Dorset man from the county town of Dorchester, the youngest son in the family of William Treves, a well-to-do furniture salesman and upholsterer. William Treves kept a large town house above his shop, which stood in one of the main streets of the town. It was there, at 8 Cornhill, on 15 February 1853, that Frederick Treves was born.

Little is recorded of his early life. At the age of seven his education began at the small Dorchester school where his brothers were taught before him. The headmaster was the Reverend William Barnes (1801–86), a formidable scholar and linguist who was also a dialect poet of sensitivity and a figure of more than regional importance in English literary history. Both Gerard Manley Hopkins and Thomas Hardy acknowledged a debt to his influence in their poetry.

When he was writing the Dorset volume for the *Highways and Byways* topographical series on the English counties, Treves remembered the extraordinary range of his old master:

> He was familiar with all European languages . . . He could read Hindustani, Persian, Arabic and other unwonted tongues. He was a very accomplished musician, playing himself the flute, the violin, and the piano. He wrote innumerable books besides his well-known poems, and was learned in

geology and archaeology. More curious still, he was a competent engraver on both wood and copper, so that he illustrated not only his own works ... but also the books and monographs of his friends.

Treves was only at William Barnes's school for two years, but the impression left on him by this Dorset genius, who managed to combine an austere and rigorous regard for learning with a broad humanity and a delicacy of vision, was life-long. When he entered school, Treves told his publisher Newman Flower many years later, he 'was very frightened by the austere figure in black, sitting there like some grim Inquisitor in the high chair'. Mary Hardy, Thomas Hardy's younger sister who was also a pupil at the school, remembered Treves as a shy and even timid child who would, the moment lessons were over, run to hide in the cloakroom behind the coats of the other pupils until the family maid came to escort him home. Despite all this, Treves wrote that his recollection of Barnes was:

... that of the gentlest and most kindly of men. His appearance was peculiar. He had white hair and a long white beard, and always wore knee breeches and shoes with large buckles. Out of doors he donned a curious cap and a still more curious cape, while I never saw him without a bag over his shoulder and a stout staff. During school hours he was in the habit of pacing the room in a reverie, happily oblivious of his dull surroundings. I remember once that some forbidden fruit of which I was possessed rolled across the schoolroom floor, and that I crawled after it in the wake of the dreaming master. He turned suddenly in his walk and stumbled over me, to my intense alarm. When he regained his balance he apologized very earnestly and resumed his walk, unconscious that the object he had fallen over was a scholar. I have often wondered to which of his charming poems I owed my escape from punishment.

In due course, when he was eleven, Treves was sent to London, where his father had enrolled him at the Merchant Taylors' School. He stayed at Merchant Taylors' until he was eighteen, but as a scholar seems to have left an undistinguished record. It was only in sports, and in football in particular, that he excelled, and holidays were always a time of happy return to his home county. Throughout his later life he was to speak with deep nostalgia of the region he called 'the Dorset beyond the hills'.

It was decided eventually that he should follow his eldest brother, who had been a medical student at St Thomas's Hospital, into the medical profession. For the youngest Treves boy, though, a place was sought at the Medical School attached to the London Hospital. It was perhaps an unexpected choice. Of all the hospitals in London which then had medical schools attached to them, the London Hospital was generally considered to be the least attractive.

First and foremost there was its geographical situation. While it could claim at this time to be the largest hospital in England, it was set in the midst of the poorest large population in the country. Its 690 beds drew patients from a maze of alleys, courts and back streets that stretched along the river behind the wharfs and docks of the lower Thames. It was, after all, *the* hospital of London's East End. Patients would arrive on handcarts from the markets of Billingsgate, on stretchers from as far away as Tilbury Docks and from every noisome rat-infested slum between. The poverty of the area, the overcrowding and dirt, were almost indescribable. Portman Square off Orchard Street, for example, was a small court twenty-two feet wide with a common sewer running down the middle. Yet it served twenty-six three-storeyed houses and almost a thousand people regarded the square as home. In Wapping, the courtyards were deep in filth, and the children, often virtually naked, would crawl to search for vegetable parings in the refuse. The Thames itself, which had become the great sewer for the entire metropolis, was so offensive that Members of Parliament at Westminster complained they could not use the room overlooking the river.

The London Hospital could therefore claim to have no shortage of good clinical material on its doorstep, but it was still hardly surprising if many students coming down from Oxford or Cambridge preferred to go to some other hospital to complete their studies. If the surroundings were depressing, however, the opportunity was there to study under some of the greatest medical names of the day. The teachers included such men as Jonathan Hutchinson, a tall bearded surgeon who excelled in every field of medicine and who made so many original observations that his name is still to be found in modern textbooks of surgery; Hughlings Jackson, a brilliant and eccentric physician who has come to be recognized as one of the founders of neurology; Langdon Down, a specialist in the problems of mental deficiency who first recognized the existence as an entity of mongolism (now known more correctly as Down's syndrome); and Andrew Clark, a doctor remembered not so much for his contributions to medical science as for the fact that he was chosen as personal physician by members of the royal family and by the Liberal prime minister, W. E. Gladstone. The young Robert Louis Stevenson travelled from Edinburgh to London to consult Clark about the condition of his tuberculous lungs.

For the students, work at the London seems to have been haphazard and largely unsupervised, but its basis was unremittingly practical. Their help was necessary to cope with the scrimmage of patients who came in through the hospital doors like a tide continually on the flood. In 'The Old Receiving Room', a companion essay to 'The Elephant Man', Treves left a series of vivid vignettes of the mêlée of human distress that was likely to gather in the casualty department in his student days, when the cry that went up in the event of an accident in the London streets was not yet, 'Call for an ambulance!' but still, 'Send for a shutter!'

The receiving unit consisted first of the hall, which served as waiting room and where there could always be someone waiting:

> It may be a suffering woman who has called for her dead husband's clothes. It may be a still breathless messenger with a 'midwifery card' in her hand, or a girl waiting for a dose of emergency medicine. There may be some minor accident cases also, such as a torn finger, or a black eye like a bursting plum, a child who has swallowed a halfpenny, and a woman who has been 'knocked about cruel', but has little to show for it except a noisy desire to have her husband 'locked up'.

Then, on either side of the hall, were two dressing-rooms, assigned respectively to men and women, where surgeons and dressers worked on the emergencies on a wide couch, sinisterly covered in thick, black and much-washed leather.

It may be a man ridden over in the street with the red bone-ends of his broken legs sticking through his trousers. It may be a machine accident, where strips of cotton shirt have become entangled up with torn flesh and a trail of black grease. It may be a man picked up in a lane with his throat cut, or a woman, dripping foul mud, who has been dragged out of the river.

Finally, there were the solemnly silent processions that accompanied every street casualty all the way to the hospital gates in the days before the introduction of ambulances, any diversion from life's hard routine no doubt being more than welcome.

It is a closely packed crowd which moves like a clot, which occupies the whole pavement and oozes over into the road. In the centre of the mass is an obscure object towards which all eyes are directed. In the procession are many women, mostly with tousled heads, men, mostly without caps, a butcher, a barber's assistant, a trim postman, a white-washer, a man in a tall hat, and a pattering fringe of ragged boys . . .
The object carried would be indistinct, being hidden from view as is the queen bee in a clump of fussing bees. Very often the injured person is merely carried along by hand, like a parcel that is coming to pieces. There would be a man to each leg and to each arm, while men on either side would hang on to the coat. Possibly some Samaritan, walking backwards, would help hold up the dangling head. It was a much prized distinction to clutch even a fragment of the sufferer or to carry his hat or the tools he had dropped.

In fact the busy unsupervised atmosphere at the London Hospital seems to have suited Treves exactly. He began to display a determinedly practical approach to the problems he encountered. The firm decisions and decisive actions inherent in the surgical approach to patients seemed ideally suited to his personality, and it was to this branch of medicine that he found himself increasingly attracted.

After four years at the London Hospital, Treves's studies were completed, and in 1874, at the age of twenty-one, he took the diploma of the Society of Apothecaries. The following year he passed the examination to become a member of the Royal College of Surgeons. He then undertook a term of duty as a house surgeon at the London Hospital to build on his experience before accepting an offer from his elder brother, who was now honorary surgeon to the Royal National Hospital for Scrofula at Margate, down in Kent. There, though it was only to be for a few months, Frederick Treves became resident medical officer. Even in this brief period he managed to apply himself to an intensive study of scrofula, then still a disease of unknown origin.

By 1877 he felt the time had arrived for him to try his hand at general practice. It was a difficult time in which to start such a career, capital being necessary either to buy a share in a practice or simply to support a young doctor as he built up a practice of his own. There were also many young doctors competing for the patronage of those wealthy patients who made such a career possible and profitable. At this point Treves married Anne Elizabeth Mason, the youngest daughter of a Dorchester merchant. She brought some private money to their marriage, and it was probably this which enabled the young couple to set up home in the small town of Wirksworth, Derbyshire. Here Treves bought his way into a partnership in an isolated community, set in one of the beautiful Derbyshire vales. The practice extended for many miles to take in neighbouring farms and villages. It looked as though a dream had been realized.

In the event the idyll did not last. Treves's strong personality and the impression of confidence he conveyed to the patients precipitated jealousies among his senior partners. Within a year he was back near London, attempting to set up in general practice in the suburb of Sydenham. When, in 1878, the chance presented itself of filling the post of surgical registrar at the London Hospital, the opportunity seemed too good to miss. This relatively humble post was to provide the springboard for his whole future career.

The rungs of the ladder that Treves now mounted were placed as follows. First, in 1879, he became assistant surgeon to the London Hospital, and shortly afterwards also an assistant at the Royal

London Ophthalmic Hospital. This led to his being made lecturer and demonstrator in anatomy to the London Hospital Medical School, a position he used to pioneer research in the whole new range of abdominal operations that anaesthesia and new antiseptic techniques were making possible. His research notes from his work on scrofula provided him with the material for his first book, *Scrofula and Its Gland Diseases* (1882).

Treves was now able to live up to the aspiration of owning a home in Bloomsbury, where he occupied 18 Gordon Square with his wife and two baby daughters. Other honours and publications followed, and he found he could only get through all his commitments by observing a stringent self-discipline, rising as early as five or six each morning to write, study or catch up on correspondence before proceeding to his main duties of lecturing and operating throughout the day in the Medical School. The surgeon's task was heavy and exacting. One house governor of the London Hospital recalled how Treves's operating coat became so stiff with congealed blood that it stood upright without visible means of support when placed on the floor.

Already Treves had developed the combination of brusque directness and glimpsed moments of bluff yet genuine kindness the public mind associates with eminent physicians. He became immensely popular with many of his students, to whom he preached a message of self-reliance: that they should rely on their judgement, make a firm decision and unhesitatingly act on it. The student who said to him one day about a case, 'It might be a fracture, sir, or it might be only sprained,' was sharply rebuked: 'The patient is not interested to know it might be measles or it might be toothache. The patient wants to know what is the matter, and it is your business to tell him or he will go to a quack who will tell him at once.'

Despite his many professional duties, he still found time to speak for the Temperance Society on 'Alcohol: a Poison'; and to become chairman of the medical section of the Mission to Seamen. Then, with the year 1884, he was elected to the position of full consulting surgeon to the London Hospital.

Another change of life-style became necessary. He now had to build up a private consulting practice to bring him fees to make up for the fact that this was no salaried post, though he would continue to receive fees for his teaching and he had, of course, royalties from his published writings. Promptly he moved his family from Bloomsbury to 6 Wimpole Street, where he was able to set up consulting rooms in the heart of the Harley Street area.

It was a period of industrial depression, when few working-class families had as much to live on as £1 10s. (£1.50) a week. Yet, as Treves knew, at least one of his colleagues at the hospital, Sir Andrew Clark, was earning over £12,000 a year. 'Considering the number of patients who can comfortably be seen between nine and two o'clock and the number of visits that can be managed between two and seven,' Sir Andrew once wistfully remarked, 'I see no hope of improving that figure.' On the other hand, income tax had just been reduced from 8d. to 7d. in the pound.

The world, in a very real sense, was on the verge of opening out at Treves's feet. And this was precisely the stage his life had reached on the day when Dr Tuckett told him about the very odd Elephant Man to be seen in a freakshow across the road from the London Hospital, and was persuasive enough to make him decide to go and take a look.

CHAPTER 3

A Living Specimen

Eventually they stood facing each other in Treves's room in the Anatomical Department of the Medical School of the London Hospital.

We cannot begin to guess at what the freak from the exhibition shop made of Frederick Treves, this tall young surgeon, broad-shouldered and athletic in build, intensely observant and self-assured, possessing indeed a master's sailing certificate for his recreational yachting activities on the Dorset coast; a man who had already witnessed in his professional life most of the varieties of disease and physical distortion induced by environment, behaviour or genetic misfortune in the slums of the world's greatest metropolis, but who had never come across anything quite like the Elephant Man before.

By contrast, we know what Frederick Treves made of Joseph Merrick as he measured him up and stripped him finally naked to the point where he was fully revealed as the most bizarre spectacle imaginable. Yet, of the man himself, he says little. 'He was shy, confused, not a little frightened and evidently much cowed. Moreover, his speech was unintelligible . . . I supposed that Merrick was imbecile and had been imbecile from birth.' The emphasis of the examination was on the physical aspects: to pass a tape measure round the head and limbs, finger the skin, assess the movement of the joints, hold back the shapeless blubber of the lips with a spatula to examine the inside of the mouth. There were massive abnormalities of the skin and flesh as well as some obvious and extraordinary distortions in bone structure. Meticulously Treves charted every feature, recorded each peculiarity that he could discover on the appalling map of Merrick's body, but seemed to have hardly begun to approach any closer to an explanation in this chaotic anatomical wilderness.

The proportions were grotesque: a measurement of 36 inches was recorded for the head's circumference, another of 12 inches for that of the right wrist and one of 5 inches for the most swollen finger of the right hand. Yet Merrick was a short man, scarcely more than 5 feet 2 inches in height. In the skin Treves felt he could recognize two distinct abnormalities. First, there was an abnormality of the soft, subcutaneous tissue that lay immediately beneath the skin. It seemed in places to have greatly increased in quantity so that in these regions the skin was raised up above the surrounding tissue. Where this happened, the skin was so loose on the body that it could be slipped about quite easily, or grasped and drawn away from the deeper tissue in folds.

In three areas these changes were so marked that the weight of the skin drew the tissues down into pendulous folds that hung almost like curtains of flesh from the body. One of these folds, about six inches square, hung in front of the right armpit, taking its root from the surface of the right breast and shoulder. A similar but less conspicuous fold hung down behind the armpit. It was in the buttocks, however, that the process was most marked. Here the skin flap was so thick and extensive that at first sight it looked as though the buttocks themselves descended in a great fold reaching almost to the level of the mid-thigh. So heavy and awkward was this fold of flesh that it tended to interfere with the functioning of the bowel and the action of defecation.

The second abnormality Treves recognized in the skin was the presence of numerous warty growths or papillomata. These varied in size from small pimple-like roughenings of the skin to huge cauliflower-textured masses. Their size and number varied between different areas of the body. In fact, the skin of the left arm was free from blemish, and parts of the face, and the eyelids and ears, seemed unaffected; the penis and scrotum were perfectly normal. Over the chest and abdomen the warts were small and sparse, but over the back of the head, and from between the shoulder blades down to the lower back and buttocks, they spread out as exuberant growths of dusky purplish skin, deeply cleft and fissured. From the largest of these warty growths there rose the exceedingly foul odour that Treves first noticed in the exhibition shop.

If the skin changes made Joseph hideous, however, it was the skeletal changes which made him misshapen; but again, not all of the body was affected. Metamorphoses in the bones seemed to be confined to the skull, the bones of the right arm and hand and those of each leg below the knee.

The skull was enormous. It was completely irregular in shape, its surface being covered by huge rounded bosses of bone, some of them larger than tangerines. The most conspicuous bony lump stood out on the brow, but there were others to the side and back of the head. The whole left side of the head actually seemed to bulge out immediately above the ear, so that the ear was itself folded downwards almost at a right angle. It was extremely difficult to trace the complete surface of the skull with any precision, for over most of the scalp the skin had produced cauliflower-like masses and folds of loose skin in abundance.

The bones of the face were similarly distorted. The forehead was unduly large, uneven and rather protuberant, making the eyes appear small and set back deeply in the head. The bones of the right cheek were also much enlarged, so that the cheek was hard and prominent. The swelling here had pushed the hard palate forward and down and forced the nose and mouth somewhat to the left. When the mouth was open it was possible to see a scar where a piece of tissue had evidently been removed at some time by an operation; the lower jaw seemed quite normal.

The right arm was greatly inflated, being two or three times the size of its fellow. Treves gained the impression that every bone in the limb, apart from the shoulder blade and collar bone, was uniformly enlarged, but there were none of the knobbly swellings upon the bones that were so prominent in the skull. The fantastic distortions of the bones had almost crippled the arm, for when Treves tried to manipulate it he found that, while it could be moved fairly freely at the shoulder and elbow, the wrist and fingers were so stiff as to make the hand almost useless. Merrick could not, for example, turn this particular hand over and back again. The hand meanwhile was weirdly deformed, its huge misshapen fingers crowding one another into deformity and even partial dislocation of the joints. Strangely enough, though, the finger nails on the hand were perfect. As if in mocking contrast, the left arm was completely unaffected, having a delicacy and neatness of proportion that made Treves think of the arm of a young girl.

Both feet were distorted in a manner similar to the right arm, the bones being uniformly enlarged and the toes malformed and enormous. Merrick's posture illustrated the presence of the old disease of his left hip that Treves had already diagnosed, for he stood with his left leg held stiffly forward and away from the body. Apart from the tell-tale sign of a former hip disease and the various changes to the skin and bones, however, Treves could find little else amiss. The irony was that the Elephant Man apparently enjoyed good health in all other respects, suffering from no serious illness apart from his mysterious condition and even possessing an appreciable muscular strength.

As the examination and interview proceeded, so Treves became more accustomed to the Elephant Man's distorted fluting voice and was able to add a little to his background knowledge of the man. The operation to the upper jaw, he gathered, had been carried out a year or two earlier in Leicester Infirmary. A developing tumour of the connective tissue in this area had apparently grown to the extent where it projected so far beyond the mouth that Merrick could no longer close his lips or masticate or move his jaw effectively. The surgeons at Leicester therefore advised him that it should be cut away.

Treves tried to discover whether there was any evidence for similar deformities occurring in Merrick's family. Apparently there were none. Merrick stated that he had neither brother nor sister. His head, right arm and feet had been badly deformed for as long as he could remember, but when he was a child his skin was no more than roughened, loose and rather thick. The story of the profound shock suffered by his mother when bowled over by a circus elephant was once more offered as a helpful clue.

In writing 'The Elephant Man' Treves conveys the impression that once he had completed his examination he returned Merrick to the care of the showman at the end of the day and that was the last he saw of him during the present stage of the story. Again this is a simplification of events for he certainly remained in touch with Joseph Merrick and Tom Norman over several days. Some time during this period, if not during the initial clinical interview, he arranged for the first photographs to be taken. He also persuaded Mr Norman to allow his charge to be brought as a case for discussion and diagnosis before the eminent members of a learned medical society, the Pathological Society of London.

It seems reasonable to speculate that there would at this point have awakened in poor Joseph Merrick's heart, if not the wild hope of a cure, at least the chance of a wise, informed explanation or an assurance that something might be done to halt the encroachments of his disease.

Meetings of the Pathological Society of London were held on alternate Tuesday evenings at 8.30, at the headquarters of the society at 53 Berners Street, in Bloomsbury. Advance notice of meetings was always given in the *British Medical Journal*, together with a list of cases to be presented; it was also usual for a summary of any meeting to appear in the journal's following issue.

The *British Medical Journal* for 29 November 1884 was already in the press with its notice of the next meeting on Tuesday, 2 December, and the seven items listed for exhibition. Mr Frederick Treves was down simply to display two cases of tumour of the palate. He must have moved quickly, uncertain about how long he could remain effectively in touch with a case as peripatetic as a travelling freakshow exhibit. He sought and gained permission to display Joseph as an additional item at the 2 December meeting.

The Pathological Society of London was a highly respected institution. It had been in existence for thirty-eight years and was to flourish through to 1932, when it voluntarily disbanded so that it might be reconstituted as the Pathological Section of the present Royal Society of Medicine. It drew members not only from among London pathologists, surgeons and physicians, but also from doctors who worked in many of the leading provincial medical centres. A number of the society's members were not only eminent in the field of medicine but were also associated with the realms of biology and the related sciences.

On 2 December Joseph Merrick was duly conveyed during the evening from Whitechapel to Bloomsbury. It must have surprised him to find himself the only living exhibit presented, or, for that matter, the only complete exhibit in the lecture room. All the other displays consisted merely of organs or sections of tissue removed from patients during an operation or at a post mortem.

Joseph's appearance as he entered certainly caused a stir among the society's members. The most astonished of them was John Bland-Sutton, the assistant surgeon from the Middlesex Hospital who had chanced on the Elephant Man's freakshow before Treves.

> My surprise was great [he wrote] a fortnight later to find this man exhibited by Treves at the Pathological Society of London. He not only submitted Merrick for examination by members of the Society, but published a detailed and illustrated account of this unfortunate man in the *Transactions* for 1885.

Could there be just a hint in this comment that Bland-Sutton felt Treves was being a little theatrical in his choice of a case; that it lay perhaps on the borderline of medical discretion to have put it forward; that there was maybe even a touch of the showman's instincts in the action?

Yet while the Elephant Man may have been seen in his freakshow by other gifted medical personalities, the fact remains that it was Treves who took the initiative in deciding that here was a case which demanded an explanation. In fact, apart from the first murmurs of surprise, there seems to have been little response from the members. No one came forward with any constructive suggestion, and the problem of diagnosis was carried no further. The digest of the meeting that appeared in the *British Medical Journal* for the following week simply stated:

> *Congenital Deformity* – MR TREVES showed a man who presented an extraordinary appearance, owing to a series of deformities: some congenital exostoses of the skull; extensive papillomatous growths and large pendulous masses in connection with the skin; great enlargement of the right upper limb, involving all the bones. From the massive distortion of the head, and the extensive areas covered by papillomatous growth, the patient had been called 'the elephant-man'.

The correspondent for the *Lancet* evidently shared Bland-Sutton's reservations over the propriety of demonstrating such a sensational case before the society. A lengthy account of the meeting that the journal published contains no mention whatsoever of Joseph's presence.

It seemed as if Treves was fated to be left with his original vague diagnosis of a congenital deformity, and that Joseph, none the wiser for his brief sojourn among higher medical authorities, must return to the care of Mr Tom Norman and the relentless round of earning his living on the freakshow circuits. For most doctors that would have been the end of their attempts to solve such a puzzle; but Frederick Treves lacked nothing in determination. Four months later he tried again. It seemed to him just possible that, by putting the case forward one more time, having given adequate notice in the medical journals, some doctor or specialist with knowledge of such a strange condition might be encouraged to attend the meeting; or, alternatively, that the lapse of time might have allowed some of those who saw Joseph Merrick previously to consider the problem at leisure.

By now Treves knew nothing of the whereabouts of Merrick, but he had the photographs and he had the data and clinical findings from his first examination. These he was able to present to the meeting of the Pathological Society of London which was held on Tuesday, 17 March 1885. On this occasion his endeavours attracted a response. Among those gathered for the meeting was Dr Henry Radcliffe Crocker.

Radcliffe Crocker was then just forty years old, a physician from University College Hospital, London, who had specialized in diseases of the skin. As a student he had come under the influence of the late Dr Tilbury Fox, a dermatologist who attempted to reduce the then chaotic problems of dermatology to some semblance of scientific order. Tilbury Fox soon infected the younger doctor with an enthusiasm for his speciality, and within a few years Radcliffe Crocker was emerging as one of the world's leading authorities on skin diseases.

Having listened to Treves's presentation of the Elephant Man's case in silence, Radcliffe Crocker rose to make his own observations. His dissertation was quietly brilliant. Surely, he suggested, this was no new or undescribed disease. It seemed a case that must surely be classified as belonging to a rare group of disorders termed as *dermatolysis* (a loosened or pendulous condition of the skin) and *pachydermatocoele* (a condition where tumours arise from an overgrowth of skin). Both these skin disorders, though excessively rare, had been known for some years.

It was Radcliffe Crocker's opinion that these two forms of skin disorder were in some way related, that an association was already recognized between them by the medical profession; for, on one or two other occasions, as in Treves's case, they had been found to coexist in the same patient. He felt that the particular interest in the example of the Elephant Man lay in the fact that he presented a third feature: a deformity of the bones. The combination of the skin conditions with bone changes was, so far as he knew, something never before described.

Having linked three pieces in the bizarre medical jigsaw, Radcliffe Crocker rounded off his remarks with an inspired suggestion. He reminded the meeting of a case presented before the society by his old mentor, Dr Tilbury Fox, where a patient with the symptoms of a looseness of the skin had developed these after an injury and a resulting abscess that needed to be lanced. It was found that the parts of the body affected were those supplied by the nerves damaged by the injury and the subsequent abscess. Might it not therefore be that changes in the nervous system had governed the bodily distribution of the disease in the Elephant Man?

As a surmise it was still vague enough, and it still left many questions unanswered, but with the hindsight of more than a century it is possible to say it was a better explanation than Treves had a right to expect. The Pathological Society of London and Dr Radcliffe Crocker had provided as accurate an answer as it would have been possible to give anywhere in the world in the state of medical knowledge in 1885.

What, meanwhile, of Joseph Merrick and Tom Norman? The tide of rational decency was by now running heavily against their mutual interest. Even in the East End of London a new sensitivity in public opinion was leading to demands for official action to shut down exhibitions found by a growing number of citizens to be offensive. It was all part of a long and undeniably civilizing process. The 'taste for Monsters' which, Henry Morley wrote, 'became a disease' during the heyday of Bartholomew Fair, was one 'of which the nation has in our own day [the 1850s] recovered with a wonderful rapidity'. During Queen Anne's reign, at the house next to the Greyhound Inn during Bartholomew Fair, there was an exhibition of a hydrocephalic child: 'but Thirty weeks old, with a prodigious big head, being above a yard about, and hath been shown to several Persons of Quality'. There can be few societies today in which an attempt to put on such an exhibition would be greeted with anything but outrage.

Nevertheless there are always two sides to a question whenever righteous indignation succeeds in imposing its general will. In his book *The Travelling People*, Duncan Dallas records the lamentation of a post-Second World War fairground showman who was having much difficulty in finding an adequate supply of human freaks. He blamed it on the Welfare State in Britain: '... you never hear anything about these people. They seem to be smothered. They seem to be kept out of the way in the background.'

The inference is that freaks still exist in plenty but that society would prefer to avoid the discomfort of knowing about them. The old showmen, Tom Norman among them, were predictably at one in claiming that their freaks were better off out in the world, among people and earning a living, than shut away in an institution or an isolated home from which they could never venture forth, dependent on charity or welfare. So where was the line to be drawn between an object of legitimate curiosity and an offence to public decency?

There was no doubt in the minds of the London police that Joseph Merrick fell firmly within the latter category. They had therefore stepped in to close down the show in the Whitechapel Road as they would, three years later on the same site, close down the waxworks exhibition on the theme of the Jack the Ripper murders. Joseph had retreated back along the road out of the metropolis and disappeared somewhere into the provincial background. Frederick Treves had no reason to think he might ever have dealings with him again.

Meanwhile there were his notes and data as well as the photographs, and there was one further task he intended undertaking. This was to prepare his account of the case for publication in the

Transactions of the Pathological Society of London. Copies of the photographs were sent to Messrs F. Huth, Lithographers, of Edinburgh, and eventually the finished plates, together with Treves's description, were published in the *Transactions* for 1885 under the heading, 'A Case of Congenital Deformity'.

Thus Treves had made a permanent record of the case to be bequeathed to medical posterity and taken up by any future experts who might feel drawn to unravelling its mysteries. By this time he was busily engaged in delivering the Hunterian Lectures on Anatomy to the Royal College of Surgeons, and if he thought further of the Elephant Man it was to hope that his impression of him as a retarded individual was accurate.

> The fact that his face was incapable of expression, that his speech was a mere spluttering and his attitude that of one whose mind was void of all emotions and concerns gave grounds for this belief. The conviction was no doubt encouraged by the hope that his intellect was the blank I imagined it to be.

The possibility that Joseph Merrick might after all have any realization of the dilemma of his life would, Treves felt, be too appalling even to consider.

CHAPTER 4

A Parade of Elephants and Early Griefs

What therefore is known or may be discovered of the origins of Joseph Merrick?

His birth certificate gives the information that he was born Joseph Carey Merrick on 5 August 1862 at 50 Lee Street, Leicester; that his father was Joseph Rockley Merrick, warehouseman, and his mother Mary Jane Merrick, née Potterton. As the date of their marriage in the parish church of Thurmaston was 29 December 1861, it is fair to assume that Mary Jane was already pregnant by the time she went to the altar. She was twenty-six years old when she gave birth to Joseph, and his memory of her was, as we shall see, one of the most important elements in his life.

An anonymous article on the Elephant Man that appeared in the *Illustrated Leicester Chronicle* on 27 December 1930, which is clearly based on a knowledge of the Merrick family circumstances, states that Mary Jane was herself a cripple. She was born in the small village of Evington on the south-east outskirts of Leicester, the third child in a family of nine. Her parents, William and Elizabeth Potterton, were ordinary country people. Indeed, her father, a farm labourer, could not write his own name, but the Pottertons did well by their children, allowing them to attend school until they had received at least a basic education.

When Mary was about five years old her family moved from Evington to settle in the village of Thurmaston, a few miles to the north of the city. From there, at the age of twelve, she left home to become a servant to a family in Leicester itself.

For the next thirteen years she remained in service, enduring a life that could have been distinctive only for its long hours and attic bedrooms, the endless carrying of hot-water jugs and coal buckets, incessant scrubbing and blackleading and the invariable rules about 'no followers'. Then in 1861, when she was twenty-five, she met Joseph Rockley Merrick, who was just over a year younger than herself. He made his living as the driver of a brougham, a closed four-wheeled cab.

The Merrick family's village of origin is reputed to be Clynnogfawr in North Wales, but by the 1780s they were established in London. Joseph Rockley Merrick's father Barnabas (the third Barnabas running in order of descent) had been born in 1792 at Spitalfields, where the family was successful in the weaving trade, owning looms, engines to run them and leasehold property. He married, first, in 1815, a bride from Wanstead, who bore him four children, and secondly, in 1826, a Sarah Jones, though this marriage was childless. By the 1830s he was working as a bobbin-turner in the hosiery trade in Leicester, and in 1837 he married for the third time, to Sarah Rockley from Radford in Nottinghamshire.

Joseph Rockley Merrick was the eldest of Barnabas and Sarah's three sons, the other two being Henry and Charles Barnabas Merrick, all born in Leicester. After Joseph Rockley and Mary Potterton had married in turn, they set up their first home at 50 Lee Street, a small house in one of the warren of streets behind Humberstonegate, only a few yards from the address of Joseph Rockley's by then widowed mother Sarah.

The city of Leicester was meanwhile expanding rapidly on the basis of the industrialization of its traditional crafts of hosiery and knitwear, to which were added boot and shoe manufacture. Fresh mazes of narrow streets and dingy back-to-back housing sprang up with regularity in each succeeding year. From the north side of Humberstonegate a long, narrow street called Wharf Street ran down at right angles to reach the new public wharf on the canal. The land to each side of Wharf Street was low-lying, even marshy, but by the 1860s the gardens and nurseries still charted on the maps of 1828 had disappeared beneath a confusion of backstreets. Lee Street was one of these: a side-turning off Wharf Street.

From its moment of construction Lee Street could justly be defined as a slum. The houses were small and lacked running water. Sanitation was a constant problem, for the sewers were inadequate and many houses possessed only cesspits. The removal of refuse was in the hands of private scavengers who were both ineffective and irregular. Worst of all were the floods. Once a year the River Soar and the canal could be expected to rise and fill the streets to a depth of two or three feet, the water having forced its way back up through the sewers, bringing with it sewage and garbage. It was both insanitary and lethal. Over many years Leicester suffered a death-rate that annually removed between twenty-six and thirty in every thousand of its population; and, as always, the death-rate was highest among infants and children. The Victorian mothers of the time had little hope of being spared the helpless despair of watching at least one of their children sicken and die.

Shortly after his marriage Joseph Rockley Merrick changed his job, giving up his employment as a brougham driver and going to work in one of the many cotton factories. The work was monotonous and the hours were long, the usual shift lasting from 8 a.m. to 7 p.m. in winter and from 6 a.m. to 5.30 p.m. in summer, with half an hour for breakfast and dinner. Many firms by this time allowed Saturday afternoon as a half-day off, but there were no statutory bank holidays and even Boxing Day was regarded as a normal day of work. Wages varied, but a man working two knitting frames could earn as much as 12s. (60p) or 15s. (75p) a week, a woman 9s. (45p) and even a child might bring home 2s. (10p) or 3s. (15p). Joseph Rockley Merrick was somewhat more fortunate in that he managed to obtain a position in the warehouse where the wages were slightly higher than those paid to the operatives. Men and women who worked in the warehouse were generally regarded as a better class of employee.

In Leicester, Mary came under the influence of the Baptist ministry. This was particularly strong in the town, and for a period in her life she was a teacher in one of the three Baptist Sunday schools in the city, though which one is unrecorded. Education in Leicester, as in many of the other new and growing industrial centres, presented a considerable problem in the 1860s. Children of seven and eight years old were still being employed by cotton factories, by boot manufacturers and in the brickyards. There were no free schools prior to the Education Act of 1870, and often parents could not afford to pay even the small fees charged by the various day schools, apart from their unwillingness to sacrifice the wages of their earning children. Only a third of the children in Leicester received a full-time education, and many of these attended for such short periods that they could have gained little benefit.

For the other two thirds of the children there were the Sunday schools, usually run by the Nonconformist churches. The purpose of these was to teach not only religious instruction, but also the rudiments of reading, writing and arithmetic. While we do not know which Baptist Sunday school employed Mary, the activities of the Friar Lane Baptist Sunday School give an indication that the régime was sternly imposed alongside the benevolent motivation of the Nonconformist conscience in working for the betterment of working-class children.

The Sunday schools were often surprisingly large establishments. The Friar Lane establishment had as many as 350 pupils and 45 teachers. Admission was a matter of application and interview, and truancy led to expulsion, for discipline was strict. At the beginning of the nineteenth century this school had even possessed a pair of stocks for the correction of the unruly. Successful scholars could, however, look forward to prize day and receiving certificates of proficiency; and there was always the annual Sunday school outing.

The relentless work routine for the populace of the industrial centres of the nineteenth century created, by reaction, an appetite for diversion and cheap entertainment during those few hours people could call their own. The 1860s were the first great period of growth for the institution of the British music hall throughout the provinces, although many of the new halls continued to be attached as incidental attractions to existing inns and taverns. There were meanwhile the more traditional diversions whose origins ran far back into antiquity: the charter fairs and visiting circuses and menageries, the latter featuring elephants among their attractions. And the mention of elephants at once sets off an echo: the carefully tended story that Joseph Merrick put forward to account for his condition, that his mother had been knocked down by an elephant during the time she carried him in her womb.

The *Leicester Journal* for 9 May 1862 contained the following announcement:

Notice is hereby given that the next Leicester MAY FAIR will be held on Monday, the 12th day of May next for the sale of horses, beasts and sheep, and on Tuesday, the 13th and following days for the sale of cheese. By order, Saul Stone, Town Clerk. N.B. No cheese wagon will be allowed to enter the Market Place except from Hotel Street.

The following day the *Leicester Chronicle* dutifully repeated the notice.

There had been fairs in Leicester since the thirteenth century. The dates of the fairs, and the festivals they celebrated, had varied over the years, but gradually they coalesced into the two great annual fairs of the city. The first was held early in May each year, at the time of the 'Invention of the Cross'; the second in early October. Before their discontinuation in 1902, they were among the truly great charter fairs of Britain. People would pour into the city from the neighbouring villages and towns to buy and sell in the markets, hire employees and domestic staff and assess the quality and prices of cattle and horses. They replenished farmhouse stocks for another six months, exchanged domestic news with neighbours, bought clothes and marvelled at new fashions, pushed their way between the street stalls and ended up revelling in the tomfooleries of the pleasure fair.

For the citizens of Leicester the fairs were a mixed blessing as the streets and thoroughfares became blocked by stalls and surging crowds. Cotton spinners hurrying in the early morning to the small factories and mills would find their paths blocked by the cattle being driven through to the Cattle Market in the city centre. For two days the streets grew foul and treacherous. As Dr John Barclay of Leicester remarked in a lecture he delivered in 1864:

That the cattle market is a terrible nuisance no one will, I think, deny. I am sure that no one will say a word in support of it who have to barricade their doors against the filthy accumulations that make the streets look and smell like a cowshed for a couple of days. In my own part of the town we are quite blockaded . . .

The very next day after the cattle sales were over the poultry came into town, noisy and crowded into the backs of a hundred carts. Then there would be a day of comparative peace and cleanliness as the cheese fair took over. From every farm and dairy the great cheeses were brought, laid on fresh straw in the bottoms of carts. From end to end of the town the carts, their horses unharnessed, stood backed against the kerbs, tailboards lowered to display the cheeses to passers-by. Shopkeepers and housewives alike would move along the line, tasting samples before buying. The best cheeses went quickly to the large grocers; only the worst cheeses would still be left when the gas lamps were lit at early dusk.

In the meantime, as the trading fairs proceeded, the Humberstonegate was, as one of the wider thoroughfares of the town, set aside for the great pleasure fair. Stalls and booths were ranged down either side of the street, and where the road widened into its broadest part there were swings and merry-go-rounds; theatrical booths and marionettes; freakshows, sword swallowers and jugglers; stands for the sale of sweets, pastries and patent medicines.

Mrs I. C. Ellis, in her collection of reminiscences, *Nineteenth Century Leicester*, remembered it thus:

> The fair in Humberstonegate was a glimpse of paradise. It was a never forgotten joy to go on the roundabouts though we never ventured on the swings. The wild beast show roared and smelt like nothing else on earth, but the daintiest, loveliest thing was the marionette show. We were taken down the bazaars – and very nice the stalls were – a long row of tents with wares all on one side ... There were booths with dancers in tights disporting themselves on a platform – these our father or other conductor avoided, but the marionettes we were allowed to see ... We went to front seats (2d. by the side door, 1d. if you went in at the front, in view of all the fair). When we had all been paid for and were sitting as we thought in seclusion, the proprietor opened the front of this tent and displayed his respectable audience, and shouted again, 'Twopence in at the side door, one penny in at the front.'

In its report of the 1862 pleasure fair, the *Leicester Journal* succeeded in putting across the general aura of excitement:

Giants, descendants in direct line from the Anakims of old; india-rubber men; or acrobats; wonders of every description in animated nature, and astonishing novelties in art, are presented. A picture of a monstrous pig, exhibited outside one booth, is said to have its perfect living counterpart weighing several tons within. At another booth resides a cow, whose hind quarters are adorned with an extra leg, which the proprietor informs us, is intended expressly for scratching her nose.

The *Leicester Chronicle*, taking up the theme, adopted a more jaundiced tone:

Not withstanding the heavy showers of rain and the some-what limited attractions ... it has been visited by a large number of the country folk during the week ... There was a new circus, Croueste's, displaying to the admiring gaze of the juveniles a number of coloured vignettes, representing eques-trians in all sorts of impossible attitudes; and a dilapidated theatrical booth, with actors and actresses, whose dresses were in admirable keeping with the woe-begone appearance of the building. A giant pig, a threelegged cow, some dirty looking and rickety swingboats, really superior roundabouts, stalls for nick-nacks, and rifle galleries – made up a somewhat motley gathering of the peripatetic tradesfolk.

Yet this paragraph continues with what is, from the point of view of the present account, an intriguing snippet of information: 'The principal feature has been, of course, Wombwell's Menagerie ...' The wild-beast show could hardly fail. Permanent collections of animals were still extremely rare, so the only opportunity most people had of seeing exotic zoological specimens was offered by the travelling menageries. There were in the country several different companies on the road each year, including Atkins's and Sedg-wick's, but the most famous in the annals of fairground history was Wombwell's Royal Menagerie.

It was founded in 1807 by George Wombwell, of whom William Hone spoke ill when he encountered him at Bartholomew Fair in 1825:

... he ... exhibited himself, to my judgment of him, with an understanding and feelings perverted by avarice. He is under-sized in mind as well as in form, 'a weazen, sharp-faced man', with a skin reddened by more than natural spirits, and he speaks in a voice and language that accord with his feelings and propensities.

Hone also held against Wombwell a disgraceful event of a short while before at Warwick, where the publicity-minded proprietor set up a gladiatorial combat in which his two lions, Nero and Wallace, were baited by dogs. Despite (or because of) such episodes, Wombwell's flourished, growing ultimately into three separate touring menageries and on five occasions receiving a royal command, thrice to appear before Queen Victoria herself.

Thomas Frost, author of *The Old Showmen and the Old London Fairs*, has left a memory from boyhood of the magic anticipation Wombwell's aroused for him at Croydon Fair:

I ... could never sufficiently admire the gorgeously uni-formed bandsmen, whose brazen instruments brayed and blared from noon till night on the exterior platform, and the immense pictures, suspended from lofty poles, of elephants and giraffes, lions and tigers, zebras, boa constrictors, and whatever else was most wonderful in the brute creation, or most susceptible of brilliant colouring. The difference in scale to which the zoological rarities within were depicted on the canvas, as compared with the figures of the men that were represented, was a very characteristic feature of these pictorial displays. The boa constrictor was given the girth of an ox, and the white bear should have been as large as an elephant, judged by the size of the sailors who were attacking him among his native ice-bergs.

Elephants had a way of figuring largely in anecdotes of Womb-well's exploits. On one occasion the proprietor mistimed his tour and, Thomas Frost tells us, was still in Newcastle-upon-Tyne with only two weeks to go before the opening of Bartholomew Fair in London. The possibility of reaching London in time with his procession of caged beasts along the roads of those days therefore looked remote. At this point Wombwell gained wind of the fact that his arch-rival, Atkins, was promoting his menagerie at Bartholomew's as 'the only wild beast show in the fair'. Without hesitation Wombwell undertook a forced march to bring his caravanserai to London on the day the fair opened; but the epic effort took its toll of the elephant, the unfortunate beast dropping dead on arrival. Atkins lost not a moment in declaiming that he had 'the only living elephant in the fair'; at which Wombwell counterattacked with his slogan: 'The only dead elephant in the fair.' The tactic paid off, remarks Frost, since a 'dead elephant was a greater rarity than a live one, and his show was crowded every day of the fair, while Atkins's was comparatively deserted'.

For the Bartholomew Fair of 1830, Wombwell's proudest boast was the Elephant of Siam, 'a theatrical performer', says Henry Morley, 'in the spectacle of the *Fire-fiend*, wherein it uncorked bottles and declaimed for the Rightful Prince. On each side of it he had in his show two miniature elephants, the "smallest ever seen in Europe".'

It was a Wombwell elephant, too, that once broke out of the fairground to take a leisurely stroll down Croydon High Street in the small hours of the morning, to the alarm and bewilderment of the town constable. The animal stopped at a confectioner's, butted in the shutters and window panes with its head and helped itself to cakes and dainties.

By 1862, when Wombwell's was travelling to Leicester for the May fair in Humberstonegate, its founder had been dead a dozen years and the main company was under his widow's management. The routine leading up to the menagerie's arrival in town followed, however, a long-established pattern. First the advance agents arrived to book the site, arrange water supplies and stabling, buy in corn and forage. The printers were commissioned to run off handbills, posters went up on walls and announcements were inserted on the front pages of local newspapers whose inside columns carried news of the American Civil War.

Finally, on the first day of the fair, the city found itself aroused at seven in the morning by the rattle and shaking of a column of heavy wagons proceeding through the streets. The convoy consisted of the accommodation caravans, the provision carts and seventeen or eighteen beast wagons. These last, being cages, were eight feet high and broad and as long as eighteen feet, their occupants concealed by great shutters, their wheels iron-rimmed and noisy. Each wagon was drawn by a team of as many as four shire horses that strained before each one, their hooves slipping and sparking on the cobbles; and marching between the wagons, sometimes hitched to one or other of the larger vehicles, there walked elephants and camels.

Once in Humberstonegate, with shouting and a pushing of horses, the wagons were backed up to form a square. Three sides were formed by the wagons themselves. The fourth consisted of the high wooden façade that formed the front of the show. It was decorated with mock wooden pillars and painted panels depicting enraged beasts duelling in impossible jungles while men, magnificent in bare-chested bravery, wrestled with ferocious lions. In the centre of the façade was the pay-box, perched high on a small platform, and the square, when complete at last, was roofed over by canvas sheeting stretched from wagon to wagon. Finally, on the inside of the square, the yellow shutters of the wagons would be lowered on their hinges to mask the wheels and reveal the beasts inside.

Up the steps and past the pay-box the customer could then duck through the curtains screening the doorway to find himself at the head of the steps that led down into the covered square. Tethered here and there in small groups about the compound stood llamas and camels and other hopefully acquiescent creatures. In the cages about the square were wolves and leopards, bears, monkeys, zebras, small antelopes, parrots and pelicans. There might be a tiger, though this was a rather uncommon beast, the showmen finding tigers unpredictable and difficult to train. Two of the cages were for lions. In these a lion tamer stood face to face with two or three of the great cats, making them pose, leap through hoops, lie down and stand to command. But if the lions provided thrills, it was the elephants that imparted a feeling of solid merit to the spectacle. The local population was given to judging the status of any menagerie by the size and number of its elephants.

At midday each day it was therefore customary to open the side gates of the menagerie for the elephants to parade solemnly out and move ponderously through the streets as an impressive walking advertisement. Their procession was one of the highlights of the pleasure fair, and the reporter from the *Leicester Journal* was speaking for many when he cheerfully summed it up in the phrase that Wombwell's was here 'in all its glory'.

The reports of the local press in Leicester for May 1862 contain no mention of an unfortunate girl, crippled and pregnant, stumbling when forced by the crush of the crowd on to the roadway in front of a parading elephant, falling but scrambling clear, distressed and badly shaken. There is no reason why there should be such a record, nor any reason why anyone should have known about the incident afterwards, aside from the immediate bystanders. Yet it has become an event so inextricably intertwined in the legend of the Elephant Man, an incident so often mentioned by those acquainted with Joseph Merrick, that it would be unreasonable to suppose it never occurred.

Mary Jane Merrick gave birth to her first child three months after the Humberstonegate fair. He was christened Joseph after his father, while for a second name his mother chose Carey, calling him after the leading Baptist preacher and missionary, William Carey (1761–1834), who had done much to foster the Baptist ministry in Leicester. Carey not only founded the Baptist Missionary Society in London, but was also one of its two first missionaries. Three weeks after her son was born, Mary herself attended at the Register Office to record the birth.

To begin with, Mary and Joseph noticed no fault in their little boy. The anonymous but informative article that appeared in the *Illustrated Leicester Chronicle* in December 1930 states: '... the relatives declare ... Merrick was born a perfect baby'. He must have seemed perfectly made, even delicately proportioned, and in spite of the hazards of his environment and an epidemic of smallpox that raged through Leicester in the following year, Mary was spared the pain of losing him. He not only survived but evidently flourished for a time.

Mary's joy was, however, destined to be short-lived. Her infant son would soon start to grow grotesquely deformed, each year of his life bringing an increase of distortion and affliction. There is some confusion over how the onset of Joseph's symptoms occurred; available accounts vary greatly as to when the first manifestation of his disease became unavoidably obvious. One writer, in the *British Medical Journal* of 19 April 1890, suggested it was almost certain that the Elephant Man was born with enlargements of the bones of the skull, right arm and feet. Yet Joseph himself wrote: 'It was not perceived much at birth, but began to develop itself when at the age of five years.' Again it is to the article in the *Illustrated Leicester Chronicle* that we owe the only detailed account.

According to this, it was when her baby was about twenty-one months that Mary first became aware of something strange happening, of a firm swelling on his lower lip. During the next few months, this increased in size, spreading up as a hard tumour into the right cheek until the little child's upper lip was being pushed outwards by a mass of pink protruding flesh. Mary must have been tormented by the gradual realization that there was something seriously abnormal about her boy and that the trouble showed no sign of passing. As he grew, a bony lump appeared on the forehead, and this, too, increased in size. His skin became rather loose and rough in texture; even his bodily proportions were starting to be marred by peculiar enlargements of the right arm and each of his feet.

Among all the bizarre distortions afflicting the body of her child, the most terrible for Mary must surely have been the initial extraordinary mass of flesh that continued to force its way from beneath the upper lip. It was eventually to protrude several inches in a grotesque 'snout' weighing three or four ounces. To the most unimaginative eye, a resemblance to an elephant's trunk must have suggested itself at once. During those early years, Mary's mind doubtless went back ever more frequently to her mishap with the elephant in Humberstonegate as she cast helplessly around to explain the inexplicable – to herself as much as to her relations and gossiping neighbours.

In the meantime, Joseph Rockley Merrick had again moved house, taking his family from Lee Street to their new home at 119 Upper Brunswick Street. He had also again changed jobs. The history of the hosiery industry in the first half of the nineteenth century is the story of its mechanization. Steam power had altered the pattern of this former cottage industry and during the 1860s a social observer in Leicester counted more than 250 factory chimneys on the city skyline. Joseph Rockley's new employment was as the stoker on a steam engine in one of the cotton factories.

Shortly after moving into their new home Mary became pregnant for the second time, and on 8 January 1866 she gave birth to her second son. She called him William after her own father, and added Arthur. Any fears she may have had that her second child would develop similar deformities to those crippling her firstborn proved groundless. William Arthur's growth, it is said, remained free of abnormalities.

At about this time her elder son suffered a further misfortune. He fell heavily, damaging his left hip. After the injury the joint became diseased, and so the accident left him permanently lame. His appearance must already have been making it difficult for him to mix with other children; now it would have become impossible for him to join in their games since he could do little more than hobble. His mother no doubt did her best to ensure that his life remained as close as possible to normal, for she sent him to school each day; but she must have realized that the deformities were leaving their mark, that he was becoming a lonely introspective child, isolated from his fellows and increasingly dependent on herself for company.

On 28 September 1867 she gave birth to her third and last child. This time it was a daughter. The infant was given the Christian names of Marian Eliza, but any hopes of rejoicing at the arrival of a baby girl in the household were dashed from the start. Marian Eliza too, it seemed, carried the family curse and was born a cripple.

Joseph Rockley Merrick applied himself diligently to his work and achieved further promotion. By now he could classify himself as 'engine driver at the cotton factory'. He also threw his energies into planning a modest but independent commercial enterprise, perhaps in a desperate attempt to make a secure future for a family that had come to include three cripples. The *Leicester Trade Directory* for 1870 (prepared in 1869) lists him as proprietor of a haberdashery shop at 37 Russell Square, a small square to the north end of Wharf Street. He had never had any intention of relinquishing his job at the factory. This was one among many small 'back street' family enterprises run by wives or relatives. As such it must have been moderately successful since it continued to gain mention in the *Leicester Trade Directories* through until 1880. Meanwhile he moved his family once again, not to live in the house above the shop but to another house at 161 Birstall Street, a side street close to Russell Square.

The haberdashery shop was not long in business before even more serious personal troubles began to beset the family. In the days of preparation leading up to Christmas 1870, the Merricks' second son, little William Arthur, nearly five years old, fell dangerously ill with scarlet fever. Within twenty-four hours his condition was desperate and on 21 December he died. The following day Mary attended the Register Office to notify his death, and the death certificate bears mute witness to the devastation she felt at the loss of her one perfect child. When she came to sign the document, Mary, the Sunday school teacher who had signed her name so confidently on her own marriage certificate and each of the birth certificates of her children, could manage no more than a cross, identified by the registrar as 'the mark of Mary Jane Merrick, present at the death'.

The only prospect she had of burying her grief lay in her time-consuming round of responsibilities: two crippled children to care for and the management of the shop in Russell Square on her husband's behalf. It may be that her strength was at a low ebb by the spring of 1873 when she fell ill with bronchopneumonia. Her struggle with the disease did not last long. In the early hours of Thursday, 19 May, she died. The day was her thirty-sixth birthday, and her son Joseph was then just three months short of reaching the age of eleven.

When he wrote 'The Elephant Man', Frederick Treves, on the basis of what he knew of Joseph Merrick and his past history, reached the conclusion that Joseph's memory of his mother as a beautiful woman who had loved him was a fantasy. He thought he needed to sustain it for psychological reasons, to counterbalance his own ugliness and the fact that 'since the day when he could toddle no one had been kind to him'. Mary Jane Merrick was thus dismissed as 'worthless and inhuman', a woman who 'basely deserted' her small son and abandoned him to the workhouse. In the perspective of what is now known this may be seen as an unfortunate if unintended libel; and to be doubly unfortunate in that it posthumously compounds Mary Jane's personal tragedy.

It remains a curious fact that, during his first meeting with Frederick Treves, Joseph Merrick chose not to reveal to the surgeon certain essential pieces of information concerning his family background: that his mother had been a cripple, that he had a brother who died in early childhood, that a sister still lived who was also crippled. He never was to do so.

CHAPTER 5

The Mercy of the Parish

To be fair to Frederick Treves, Joseph Merrick could be remarkably vague about the details of his personal life. He was even uncertain over his year of birth, recording it as 1860 in the freakshop pamphlet *The Autobiography of Joseph Carey Merrick*, which is reproduced as an appendix (pages 173–5). Throughout the pamphlet the chronology is haphazard and unreliable, but we have seen that he was ten years old when his mother died from pneumonia. It was an unfortunate time of life for him to be deprived of her love and affection, though he was always to carry her in his mind as an idealized but vivid memory. The memory was of someone who had seemed the source of all the warmth and comfort he ever knew. For Joseph, the disaster marked the end of his childhood. It was, he wrote, 'the greatest misfortune of my life ... peace be to her, she was a good mother to me'.

The widower Joseph Rockley Merrick now faced several difficulties. He was left with the task of raising two crippled children while combining his duties as engine driver at the factory with running a haberdashery shop. He could not turn to his family for help. His father had died in 1856 and his mother worked in the cotton factories to make ends meet. He therefore decided to break up his home and move his family into lodgings.

He found accommodation at 4 Wanslip Street, Leicester: a little street only a few hundred yards away from where they lived previously. The landlady, Mrs Emma Wood Antill, was a twenty-nine-year-old widow with children of her own. It was to her that he therefore entrusted the care of his own son and daughter, and after a short interval there came about what may be seen as a predictable conclusion: on 3 December 1874, Joseph Rockley Merrick and

Emma Wood Antill were married in the Archdeacon Lane Baptist Chapel. Their marriage certificate describes Emma as the daughter of a gentleman.

For Joseph his father's remarriage was a further calamity. Handicapped by his distressing condition and injured hip, he now found himself living in competition with stepbrothers and stepsisters who were, he said poignantly, more handsome than himself. It was a situation that condemned him to be the odd-one-out in the new family grouping, and ultimately the family outcast. He could never succeed in gaining the affection of his stepmother, who made his life 'a perfect misery'. Whatever emotional response his father may have managed to show him in the past, within his new marriage he became decisive in rejecting his lame, ugly and embarrassing son. Most probably his protective instincts came to be centred on his crippled daughter, though there were two occasions on which his sense of duty prompted him to go out and find Joseph and bring him home after he ran away.

Yet another change of address brought the family to live at 37 Russell Square, a house attached to the haberdasher's. From here Joseph attended the newly built Board School in Syston Street until he left at the end of his twelfth year, the statutory schoolleaving age established in Britain by the Education Act of 1870. His education was considered to be complete and the time to have arrived when it was expected he would find work and start contributing to the family economy. It was Emma who was particularly insistent that he should look for work, and it was on the face of it a sensible enough attitude. Given Joseph's circumstances, however, it was to become a source of bitter and insoluble family conflict.

After a persistent search, Joseph eventually found employment at the factory of Messrs Freeman's, cigar manufacturers, of 9 Lower Hill Street. He kept his job there for the best part of two years, but by the time he was in his fifteenth year the increasing weight and clumsiness of his deformed right arm and fingers made it impossible for him to carry out the finer movements necessary to the craft of hand-rolling cigars. He was forced to relinquish his post and to enter a long period of unemployment.

Each day, as Joseph tramped about the town in search of a job to replace the one he had lost, his appearance and crippled state went steadily against him. He was becoming ever more keenly aware of the financial burden he represented to his family; he was, indeed, never allowed to forget the fact, facing the endless accusations of his stepmother that he had been idling on the streets instead of searching for employment. Often enough Emma would set his plate before him with the remark that it was more than he had earned, though the plate might be only half full. He found himself the target of sneers and jibes which wounded him so sharply that he began to avoid taking meals at home. For preference, he would limp about the streets, stifling his hunger rather than face the acid tongue of his stepmother, who made no secret of how offensive she found his presence in her household.

His father must by now have been in the uneasy and unenviable position of becoming hopelessly divided between whatever sense of duty remained towards his cruelly handicapped son, his wish to shelter his daughter and the shrill, strong-willed demands of his second wife. At least it may be said in Joseph Rockley Merrick's favour that he made one more attempt to solve the problem of employment his son faced, even if it was to be his last such effort on the teenaged boy's behalf. He obtained for him a hawker's licence from the Commissioners of Hackney Carriages, and thus Joseph, equipped with a tray of stockings and gloves from his father's shop, was sent out to peddle haberdashery from door to door.

It was by this stage too late for any such venture to succeed, if it could ever have done so. Each year that passed was seeing a steady amplification of Joseph's deformities. The mass protruding from his mouth was making his speech virtually unintelligible to strangers, and he was now so distressing a spectacle that, as he limped slowly along the streets, people would stop to turn and gaze after him. Some of the more curious might even start to follow behind, staring at him whenever he paused. Any maid or housewife who came unsuspectingly to answer the door would invariably find the sight of Joseph standing on the threshold thoroughly unnerving. He soon came to realize that people avoided answering their doors if they knew it was he who sounded their bell or rapped their knocker.

To support himself, meanwhile, he was expected to sell a set quota of goods each day. It became increasingly difficult. According to the anonymous article in the *Illustrated Leicester Chronicle*, the day inevitably came which saw his failure to sell the required quantity. Joseph, malnourished as a matter of course, spent the little money he had taken on food for himself. When he eventually returned to Russell Square he received the severest thrashing he ever was given. The blows broke more than his skin; they destroyed the last slender bonds that bound him to his father. He left the house knowing this time he would never return.

As he dragged himself about the streets of Leicester, hawking on his own account and selling whatever goods he could, buying the small amounts of food he could afford, sleeping at night in the lowest of the town's common lodging houses, he was on the verge of destitution and little more than a vagrant. His father sought him no more.

Joseph Merrick's Uncle Charles was the only member of his immediate family of whom he kept a warm recollection from this period of his life. His other uncle, Henry Merrick, had left Leicester to make a career in the army that would lead him to serve in India and elevate him to the rank of troop sergeant-major before his retirement to become a publican at Poole in Dorset in the early 1880s. Charles, by contrast, remained in the city of his birth, having taken the prudent decision to become a barber's apprentice.

An apprenticeship in barbering was a long and arduous commitment. There were the years as a lather boy, hands grown sore from rubbing lather on the sandpaper chins of customers who were shaved only every second or third day. The cut-throat razor was beyond the dexterity of many men to use on themselves and the services of a barber too expensive and time-consuming to be enjoyed more than two or three times a week.

Later, as a young assistant, he no doubt practised techniques on his brothers, besides learning the arts of hairdressing, singeing and beard-trimming. (The beard had returned to favour following a fashion set by soldiers in the Crimean War, when it had, during the winter months of the campaign, been too cold to shave.) Eventually, his apprenticeship completed, he married and in 1870, at the age of twenty-four, opened his first shop as hairdresser, tobacconist and umbrella-repairer at 144 Churchgate. It was to prove a stable soundly based business that brought security to his family and continued in Leicester for four generations.

The lives of Charles Merrick and his wife Jane had not been without their troubles. By 1877, the year in which Charles's nephew Joseph found himself virtually destitute on the streets, they had seen three of their five children die before the age of eighteen months. As soon as Charles Merrick heard about Joseph's plight he nevertheless responded directly and practically. He went out into the streets of the city to search till he found the boy, then persuaded him to return with him to the home in Churchgate above the hairdressing saloon. He and his wife would take his nephew into their home to be treated as one of their own.

Joseph continued to hawk haberdashery, but now he enjoyed at least the certainty of knowing he had a place to return to where he would receive understanding and practical support. It was a period of his life that lasted for two years which must have been years of relative happiness apart from there being no remission in the merciless advance of his symptoms. His peddling expeditions grew no easier. It became usual, whenever he ventured out, for a small crowd to collect and follow in his wake wherever he went. In the end his appearance attracted so much comment and attention that the Commissioners for Hackney Carriages, on the grounds of acting in the public good, felt obliged to take measures. When Joseph's hawker's licence came up for renewal it was withdrawn.

An arbitrary fate thus once again deprived Joseph of the means to a livelihood, and he can have had few illusions about his chances of finding any other. In his uncle's household, the extra unproductive mouth to feed that he unwittingly became placed considerable extra strains on the family finances. Besides, his Aunt Jane had in the meantime had another child who lived. Joseph could not expect to continue as such a burden in any circumstances, but this narrowed his choice of action in one direction only. He must seek the co-operation of the Poor Law authorities and apply for admission to the Leicester Union Workhouse, where his grandfather, Barnabas, had died twenty-three years before, not destitute but in one of the beds kept for terminal patients.

He spent the days over the Christmas period of 1879 with his Uncle Charles and family in the house above the shop in

Churchgate. The heartache may easily be imagined. Then, during the last few days of the Old Year, still aged no more than seventeen, he parted from the only living members of his family to have treated him with charity and decency and threw himself on the mercy of the parish.

On the first Monday after Christmas 1879, a morning uncomfortable with showers of rain and a southerly wind, Joseph Merrick presented himself to William Cartwright, relieving officer for the No. 2 area of the city. The Board of Guardians responsible for administering the Poor Law in the parishes of the Leicester Union employed two relieving officers, and Mr Cartwright was the junior of them, but his work was nevertheless responsible and difficult. He was answerable for his actions not only to the Board of Guardians who were his paymasters, but also to the law. While expenditure on relief work was stringently supervised and regulated by the board, it was the relieving officer who remained liable to be summoned to court to face charges should he commit the misdemeanour of refusing relief in a case where legal entitlement existed. Should a destitute person be denied relief and subsequently die, the relieving officer concerned could even face an indictment of manslaughter. For carrying out his duties, William Cartwright received a salary of £45 a year.

When Joseph presented himself, demonstrating his deformities and pleading an inability to work, Mr Cartwright can have found little difficulty in reaching a decision. The order authorizing Joseph's admission to the workhouse was issued. On that very same morning Joseph therefore dragged his lame leg and disconcerting body up the gentle rise of Swain Street, through the grey puddles of Sparkenhoe Street to the Leicester Union Workhouse.

The establishment stood on rising ground, on the south-eastern outskirts of the town. It consisted of a complex of large red-brick buildings, each having three or four storeys of closely spaced and small square windows. The design of the building was monotonous and nondescript in the way of the Victorian workhouse style. Only the main building, which stood immediately within the gates and was flanked by two gatehouses, possessed a touch of monolithic individuality. It presented a high façade of Victorian Gothic architecture, and its great central front door had square ornate headings.

A relatively tiny, rather quaint oriel bow-window pushed itself out from the front of the building immediately above the door, while tall thin columns of brickwork, two on either side, ascended vertically to end in little mock turrets high up amid a cluster of graceful chimneys. But the overall effect remained heavy-going, and uncompromisingly authoritarian in intention.

We can be sure the routine of Joseph's admission was a miserable enough business. Presenting his pass at the gates, he was escorted to the admission block for the ritual of registration. He gave up his clothes after the pockets had been searched, any money found in them being confiscated as a contribution to his keep. His own clothes were put away for when, if ever, he might be discharged. The workhouse clothes issued in their place were made of heavy serge or fustian, drab in colour and undistinguished in pattern so as to make it seem that the inmate wore a kind of uniform. Before he could dress in them, however, he had to undergo the ordeal of the 'hot' bath. (A Leicester journalist who once disguised himself as a tramp so as to sample the amenities of the Union ferociously recorded the bitterly cold water into which he was forced at this stage of his escapade.)

Finally an entry needed to be made in the workhouse register. This large brown book, with its list of admissions and discharges, has been preserved in the archives of the Leicester Museum, and faithfully records the admission of Joseph Merrick on Monday, 29 December 1879, giving his name and parish correctly. His year of birth is curiously given as 1861, but this, as has been seen, was a matter on which Joseph remained habitually vague throughout his life. His religion is described as 'church', his occupation as 'hawker'; the reason for admission as being 'unable to work'.

Beyond the main admission block, pathways threaded their way between tall barrack-like buildings, passing workrooms, labour yards, kitchens, storerooms, laundries until, at the very back, they opened out into the workhouse yards. Here plain wooden benches stood in the shadows of the towering building and the high encircling wall shut out all but the grey wet sky and the wind. To step through any of the doorways was to step into a world of echoing stone corridors and draughty stairways which Joseph, with his lameness, must have found hard to negotiate. There were the communal dining halls, and there were high dormitories where the beds were lined up close together, thin cotton sheets and drab blankets covering straw-stuffed mattresses. When they brought Joseph to show him his bed space, with its small locker for personal belongings, he was looking down at the only corner in the vast complex of buildings that he might call his own.

To comprehend anything of Joseph's life during his few years in the workhouse we have to understand something of the principles underlying the Poor Law administration. Workhouses were never intended to be pleasant or comfortable; they were meant to solve the problem of deciding which of those among numerous applicants for aid were genuinely in need, which were not. The Poor Law Amendment Act had proposed as an alternative to 'outdoor relief' – given as food or money and usually a matter of only a few shillings at a time – that an applicant for assistance should be offered the shelter of a workhouse. Here all his or her needs would be met, but life would be hard, regimented and in general discouraging to anyone not in a true state of destitution. For such a policy to work, the workhouse existence needed to be made at least one degree less attractive than the living conditions of the most lowly paid labourer. In many nineteenth-century parishes, rural as well as urban, such an ideal of harsh austerity must have taken some effort and application to achieve.

The Board of Guardians for the Leicester Union of Parishes first erected their workhouse in 1838, designing it to accommodate 400 paupers. Yet they remained reluctant to apply the so-called 'workhouse test' in all its severity and continued to give outdoor relief on a large scale. Unfortunately the hosiery trade on which the town depended then entered a series of depressions. Unemployment became widespread until, in one period during 1848, the board found themselves paying relief to 19,000 people out of a population of 60,000. To their horror they discovered they had disbursed over £19,000 in six months. Reluctantly the board decided to apply the 'workhouse test' more generally, but before this could come into force the workhouse itself needed to be enlarged. In 1851 it was rebuilt to accommodate 1,000 souls.

On the day when Joseph Merrick was admitted, there were 928 inmates. All were classed as paupers, but the circumstances which forced each of them into the workhouse varied greatly. Some were elderly, no longer able to fend for themselves; some were widows left without means of support; some were sick and infirm. Then there were the workmen, brought to poverty by unemployment or a sudden recession in their trade; the craftsmen forced to sell their tools before becoming eligible for admission; and the wives and children of these destitute men. Homeless unmarried mothers would also be admitted to the workhouse for their lying-in. Orphans and abandoned children, tramps and vagrants, improvident paupers, even the mentally retarded and unsound of mind also sought refuge there.

At the workhouse gates this unhappy tide of humanity was segregated into groups according to age and sex. Husbands were parted from wives, children from parents, boys from girls, toddlers from infants. Each group went into the separate blocks to live apart, work apart and exercise apart. Only at mealtimes or in chapel might there be the chance of a fleeting encounter or a few snatched words.

Joseph fell within Group No. 1, of adult males between the ages of sixteen and sixty. This was the group which most concerned the workhouse authorities: adult males who had somehow failed to support themselves. Joseph's companions were thus the broken workmen, the drunkards and dissolute, the inadequate and handicapped, the crippled and retarded. Association with the outright demented he was spared since Leicester possessed its own separate system for the insane.

His life was controlled by bells, from the waking bell as early as five or six in the morning. All other main events of the day – meals, work and rest periods – were signalled by bells. At ten in the evening the doors of dormitories were locked and gas-lamps extinguished. Inmates were forbidden to go outside the workhouse or receive visitors unless they had first obtained a written order from one of the overseers. They were allowed neither beer nor tobacco. Their food was basically nutritional, but plain and monotonous, and suffered from the usual hazards which afflict institutional cooking. There were even dishes that seemed to be inventions unique to the workhouses, such as the oatmeal gruel referred to in some establishments as 'hell-broth'. Only at Christmas was the boredom of meals temporarily dispelled. To mark the festive season the Board of Guardians at Leicester customarily issued an instruction 'that the usual Christmas dinner of beef, pork, plum pudding and beer be served to the inmates of the workhouse'.

Petty breaches of discipline were punished by restriction of diet or loss of privilege. The refractory offender, defined as one who transgressed twice within a week, might find himself confined alone for one day or two. Such serious offences as refusal to work or striking an officer of the institution could lead to an appearance before the magistrates' court and a subsequent prison term. The workhouse, indeed, lived up to its name. None was allowed to remain idle. About its grounds stood the labour yards, sheds whose interiors were divided into stalls so a man might work undisturbed by his fellows. One of the most common among a range of thankless tasks was that of oakum-picking, the beating and unravelling of pieces of old rope and rag into a loose hemp to be reused. It was awkward tiring work, made more clumsy by the fact that many of the mallets provided at Leicester had lost their handles. At the end of each work period the beaten hemp would be carefully gathered and weighed, for there was always a work quota to be accomplished. Other inmates would have to meet a quota for wood-chopping, corn-grinding or the breaking of granite into chips for use on the roads. There was also digging to be done on the workhouse allotments.

For women there was perpetual washing and cleaning, and the hours of drudgery were long. Six and a half hours of washing was considered the equivalent of picking three and a half pounds of oakum. There was also the mending and making of workhouse linen and clothing, as well as work in the kitchens and dining-rooms. For the elderly there were the duties of supervising the infants or the boys and girls, acting as helpers in the lying-in rooms or as nurses for the sick, even taking charge of the mentally retarded. For the younger children there was the workhouse school, where epidemics of minor eye infection caused the Leicester authorities recurrent concern.

Only for the infants was nothing arranged, but then, as late as 1905, a Royal Commission inspecting workhouses was distressed by the provisions it found for the care of infants in many institutions. It spoke with concern of young babies lying unchanged in cold wet cots; of babies who had no hope of getting outside into the sunlight and fresh air, the only attendant present having no means of carrying them all down several flights of stairs from the nursery to the ground floor; of the helplessness of a single attendant faced with the task of feeding a roomful of toddlers from a bowl of rice pudding while armed with only one spoon.

Yet, hard as conditions were, they provided basic standards of shelter and as often as not were comparable with the conditions of home life many inmates had known. There were even families, 'the ins and outs', who caused consternation to the administrators by seeming to flout and even exploit the whole 'workhouse test' system and to thrive on the existence. These would sign themselves in during times of need, and out again whenever there was a race meeting, fair or market in the vicinity.

At the outset Joseph Merrick endured the workhouse routine for twelve weeks. Then, on Monday, 22 March 1880, he signed himself out, putting on his own clothes again and leaving shortly after breakfast. For two days he sought work, but discovered only that his circumstances remained unchanged. On the evening of the second day he was forced to turn again to the relieving officer for help. On this occasion it was the senior relieving officer, Mr George Weston, who interviewed him and heard his case sympathetically. He was granted a further order for admission, but it was too late to return to the workhouse that night. Only on the following morning did he present himself at the gates. The same ordeal of admission and registration awaited him, though now he managed to give the year of his birth correctly, and his religion as that of his mother, 'Baptist'. The reason for admission was recorded as 'No Work'.

It had been a last hopeless protest against the inevitability of his pauperism. Now he must resign himself to this existence, to a life he would later speak of with loathing and horror. On this occasion his workhouse term was to last unremittingly a full four years. There is no knowing what humiliations he suffered, what petty tauntings his condition attracted from both staff and fellow inmates in an institution never meant to be anything but heartless.

About half-way through his workhouse years, probably in 1882, though the precise date is uncertain, an episode did occur to disrupt the institutional monotony into which his life had fallen. His deformities were still advancing and were causing him increasing distress. By the standards even of the workhouse he must have presented a remarkable sight. The mass of flesh that grew from his upper jaw, and which so resembled the trunk of an elephant, was still literally growing. It was now eight to nine inches long and forcing back his lips so that he found it difficult to eat without losing the food from his mouth. His speech was almost incomprehensible, and of all his deformities it was the mass from the upper jaw which caused him most distress. In due course he was referred to the surgeons of the Leicester Infirmary.

There were at that time three surgeons associated with the infirmary (known today as the Royal Infirmary, Leicester), the eldest of whom was Thomas Warburton Benfield, who had come to Leicester as a young man after qualifying in London in 1843. He then held various appointments and won several distinctions, working mainly for the poor in voluntary Poor Law establishments. By the early 1880s he was in semi-retirement, his successor as senior surgeon at the infirmary being Charles Marriott, whose younger colleague was Julian St Thomas Clarke. All three had distinguished themselves during their training and subsequent careers, and they were beyond question highly qualified and capable in their field.

The Leicester Infirmary was itself a good provincial hospital; its results compared respectably enough with those of other hospitals about the country, though they were still depressing enough. As the hospital records for 1882 show, for the 587 operations performed there was a loss of only twenty-three lives – but the operations listed include many such minor procedures as avulsions of toenails, incisions of abscesses, circumcisions, and amputations of fingers. By contrast, of eighteen hernias treated surgically, three died. Two years later, in 1884, there were nine cases that required the abdomen to be opened, and only five of these survived. Mr Benfield, in an address to the Midlands Branch of the British Medical Association, of which he was president, could speak proudly of a mortality rate as low as one in fourteen for operations to remove stones from the bladder, but the most routine operation still tended to be a perilous venture once the risks of haemorrhage, shock or hospital sepsis were taken into account.

It is possible that Joseph was seen by all three surgeons at the Leicester Infirmary, but no records survive to tell us which of them undertook responsibility for treating him. It was most probably Mr Marriott, since Mr Benfield was by now associated only as a consultant. At all events, Joseph was advised that something might be done to help the swelling from his mouth, provided he was willing to risk an operation. It cannot have been an easy choice given the existing hazards. At the best of times, the average expectation of life in the 1880s was still only forty-one years. Yet Joseph placed himself in the hands of the surgeons, ready to take the risks for any relief their knives might bring him. Arrangements were made for his admission.

By that time the long dark wards of the Leicester Infirmary had witnessed a century of suffering. With its 189 beds it differed little from other voluntary hospitals of the day. For support it depended on the contributions of a host of benefactors, whose names and subscriptions were carefully recorded each year in the annual hospital report. It was administered by a Board of Governors selected from among the more generous of the benefactors. Apart from accident or emergency cases, or private patients, admission could only be obtained by a letter of recommendation from a benefactor. The number of cases a benefactor might nominate in any one year was in proportion to the scale of his subscription.

The hospital wards were noisome places, with lines of low beds, each with its neat cotton counterpane. Pictures hung on the walls and the serpentine pipes feeding overhead gas-lamps ran across the ceilings. There were open fireplaces in each ward, involving the inevitable accumulations of coal dust in the hospital corridors. The centre of each ward was dominated by the ward table with bulbous brown legs and, on its surface, large winchester jars of medicine. There was the ever-present unresolved problem of fleas and bugs in the wards and cockroaches in the kitchens.

The nurses, in long dresses and starchy white aprons, stiff collars and white caps, worked long hours: as many as fourteen hours on day duty or twelve hours on nights; though two hours were free once a week, and they enjoyed one half-day and one Sunday off a month. In their first year of employment, they were paid £1 a month. Some received training, but most, particularly those of the older generation who occupied the more senior posts, had learnt their professions in a hard experience that seemed to scar their personalities with characteristic emotional toughness and cynicism.

From what is known of the hospital routine, we may reconstruct the course of events from the moment Joseph entered the operating theatre. This was a large room where everything seemed centred on the wooden table in the middle, its hinged flaps capable of being folded away from beneath any limb to be amputated. Underneath the table rested a convenient box of sawdust. There was also a black metal box in which the surgeons' instruments were stored, white china jugs to hold hot water, and the pervasive, irritating smell of carbolic spray. While the nurses continued to wear their everyday uniforms, the surgeons stood waiting in waistcoats, sleeves rolled up as they prepared to scrub hands with soap and lysol before soaking them in, first, carbolic lotion, and secondly a solution of bioiodide of mercury. It was their practice to work bare-handed.

Also awaiting Joseph was an enveloping mask of cotton gauze to cover his mouth and nose, a towel to be laid over his eyes, and then the sweet enveloping smell of chloroform and a continuing but distant sense of pain and panic.

The operation seems to have been a success, for the larger proportion of the 'trunk' on Joseph's face was removed. It can only have been a terrifying and dangerous experience, but remembering it afterwards he was able to dismiss it with the words: 'I then went into the Infirmary at Leicester when I had to undergo an operation on my face, having three or four ounces of flesh cut away . . .'

On the corner of Wharf Street and Gladstone Street, close to the Lee Street house in which Joseph was born, there stood a hotel known as the Gladstone Vaults. Its proprietor was Mr Sam Torr, whose official business was listed in the *Leicester Directory* as 'Wines and Spirits Merchant and Manufacturer of Aerated Water'. In fact he was already far better known as a star of some magnitude in the British music hall, being a figure of great popularity on the London halls, including Wilton's, where he presented his song material in the style of the *lion comique* – the song defining the character role, whether comic or sentimental, and interspersed with patter. After he had made his first fortune working the London music halls, he went to Leicester, not far from his home town of Nottingham, where his father had been a tailor, and at first became licensee of the Green Man in Wharf Street.

When he took over the Gladstone Vaults, Sam Torr certainly had his eye on its possibilities for conversion into a premises with music hall attached. His ambitions were fulfilled with the grand opening there, on 3 September 1883, of the Gaiety Palace of Varieties. Top of the bill for the opening night was Vesta Tilley, 'The Masher King ... The London Idol', and among supporting acts were Mrs John Wood, 'Nightingale of the Midlands', Mr Wilfred Roxby, 'Legitimate Character Comedian', and Messrs Young & Sandy, 'Negro Comedians'.

The hall, reported the *Nottingham Journal* on the day of the opening,

> has been converted into a spacious and excellently appointed saloon for the purpose of furnishing amusement to its frequenters. A select area near the orchestra and the chairman's seat is reserved for about fifty persons. There are seats for about 200 in the body of the hall, while a promenade gallery will accommodate a similar number. The stage is admirably arranged, and in point of tasteful decoration is scarcely surpassed by the other places of amusement in the town ... evidently no expense has been spared to render the hall as attractive as possible.

It was Sam Torr's declared intention to run his establishment along 'high class lines', seeking to cater for the 'better class society of the hosiery metropolis'. Prices for admission ranged between 6d. and one guinea. The Gaiety had as chairman Mr Will Till, himself a baritone soloist, who introduced the turns and generally presided. It also had a resident orchestra coerced into performing by a lady conductor, Mademoiselle Banvard, who rejoiced in the title of 'Leader of the Band'. Its proprietor would also not infrequently appear on his own stage to sing an item from his repertoire of comic ditties, the greatest success and constantly demanded favourite being 'On the Back of Daddy-O'. This he would perform dressed in an ingeniously devised life-size dummy with a wicker-work frame, on whose back he appeared to be sitting while it cavorted to the music. It was a droll effect that never failed.

There were six verses to the song, the first of which ran:

> Here I am, friends, how do you do,
> They call me Sam the silly-o.
> This is my old Dad you see,
> Happy, good old Billy-o.

Each verse was followed by the chorus, sung 'in quick time whilst galloping around stage':

> Gee up, gee whoa, and away we go,
> Mind yourself old laddie-o,
> Gee up, gee whoa, and away we go,
> On the back of Daddy-o.

It has been suggested that the figure of 'Daddy-o' was an early version of the ventriloquist's dummy of the later variety stage tradition, but while Sam Torr addressed remarks to it, he never made it speak in its own right. 'Daddy-o!', however, became a well-known catch-phrase of the day, and is said to have been as popular as 'By Jingo!' for a time in Victorian London.

In the meantime, the idea was taking root in Joseph Merrick's mind that the one escape route out of the workhouse open to him – the one hope he could ever have of paying his way in the world – could be to place himself on exhibition as a freak. He had heard that Sam Torr was interested in exhibiting specialities and novelties that might make a turn or display for the Gaiety. It was therefore Mr Torr to whom he wrote. The comedian responded by paying Joseph a visit in the workhouse and summing up his possibilities.

The prospect of taking on Joseph as a property certainly caught his attention, but he was too good a showman to under-estimate the complications. No exhibition featuring Joseph could hope to remain for more than a week or so in any one place before its novelty began to fade. For such a plan to succeed it was essential that arrangements be made to travel to a succession of towns. It all needed a degree of thought and organization.

Sam Torr's solution was to set about bringing together a group of businessmen with interests and establishments similar to his own. Within a short while he was able to tell Joseph that he had managed to persuade three fellow managers to come in with him to form a syndicate to organize Joseph's exhibition. As a result, on Sunday, 3 August 1884, Joseph was able to eat his last institutional breakfast, reclaim his clothes, go through the formality of obtaining a release form and turn his back on the Leicester Union and all Poor Law institutions for ever.

It was an interesting group that Sam Torr brought together to manage the promotion of Joseph's new career. Besides himself there was one other music hall proprietor: Mr J. Ellis, who styled himself 'the Caterer of Public Novelties' and owned The Living, a Palace of Varieties at the Bee-Hive Vaults, Beck Street, St Anne's Well Road, Nottingham. Another member of the group was a travelling showman who specialized in the exhibition of novelties (this rather more delicate term being preferred to 'freaks'). He was Mr George Hitchcock, known familiarly in the circles in which he moved as 'Little George'. And last though not least there was 'Professor' Sam Roper, a licensed victualler of Belgrave Gate, Leicester, who was also founder of Sam Roper's Fair, which toured regularly out of Nottingham, across into Lincolnshire and eventually to north Norfolk and King's Lynn.

Immediately after his release from the workhouse Joseph came under the care of Mr Torr and Mr Ellis. They prepared him for his first exhibition, suggesting he be presented as 'The Elephant Man, Half-a-Man and Half-an-Elephant'. So far as is known, Joseph's début before the public was at Nottingham in The Living, Mr Ellis's music hall. He was also shown in at least two other towns, including his home town of Leicester, according to one account. The time came, however, for the partnership to cast its eyes on the possibilities of London, the great metropolis, especially with the winter season approaching.

By now they were into the autumn, and George Hitchcock undertook to write to his acquaintance Tom Norman, a quick-witted young showman who was just at that time making a name for himself in the novelty display trade. Mr Norman was currently operating two show shops in the East End of London: one in Whitechapel and the other in the East India Docks Road. He replied promptly and agreed to take over the management of Mr Merrick (though in the workhouse release form he was shown he read the name as 'Meyrick'). It became Mr Hitchcock's responsibility to escort their client up to London from Leicester.

It is all too easy to see nothing but degradation in Joseph being obliged to uncover his bizarre body to public gaze and ill-informed wondering. Yet, short of a miracle, there had been no other conceivable line of escape from the grinding limbo of workhouse life in which he could only have spiralled ever downwards to an end in the unmarked shadow of a pauper's grave. Whatever humiliations fate still had in store for him, it must have been for Joseph a time of hope such as he cannot have known for many years as he took the road south to join Tom Norman in Whitechapel. It boded well to hold the key to his financial independence, the one condition that could be in harmony with his natural interior dignity. For the moment Tom Norman looked like the closest Joseph Merrick came to having a fairy godfather.

CHAPTER 6

The Silver King

Of his parents' family of eighteen sons and daughters, Tom Norman was the eldest and, as he put it himself, 'the most roving and rackety of them'. He was born Thomas Noakes at Dallington, Sussex, where his father, also Thomas, owned the Manor House with its attached farm and grazing fields and a slaughterhouse and butchers' shops. From early on he helped in his father's business, spending mornings in the shop and afternoons at the local National School. At the age of twelve he left school, and by fifteen was an accomplished butcher. He was capable of going on his own to market to select and buy cattle, afterwards driving them home to slaughter them, cut them up and sell them without further supervision.

He made his meat rounds on horseback, enlivening his days by joining up with the local hunt, the East Sussex Hounds, whenever it crossed his path, and usually leaving his meat deliveries hanging in a basket from a branch of any convenient tree. At the hunt he caught the eye of the daughter of his father's wealthiest customer and succumbed to the temptation of paying court to her. As a result his father lost trade and Tom was banned from the hunt whenever the young lady was present. In the end his father found it prudent to deny him the use of a horse whenever a hunt meeting was being held.

At seventeen Tom left home to become assistant to a butcher in London. The shop there opened at six each morning; at eight breakfast was eaten from a bench at the back; half an hour was allowed for lunch, trade permitting; and tea was a stand-up meal snatched between customers. By ten o'clock at night the working day usually drew to a close, though it might continue till midnight on Saturday. On Sunday, working hours were shorter, the shop being open only from seven in the morning till three in the afternoon. Tom Norman noted how it was the custom in town for women not to buy meat for the Sunday lunch until 1 or 2 p.m. at Sunday lunch-time. Yet, despite the long hours and hard work, he was contented, earning as much as 30s. a week with board and keep on top, and there would be a half-crown bonus in a good week.

After a year Tom temporarily abandoned the butcher's trade, determined to make a fortune by gambling on horses. After losing all his savings in the space of two days at Ascot, he abandoned the enterprise and set out to walk back to London, pausing only to ask his way from a stout gentleman whom he encountered in Windsor Great Park. A few yards further on he was accosted by an old stonebreaker at the roadside who was anxious to know what the Prince of Wales had said to him.

Back in London he settled for working at 'a large cutting butchers' in Chapel Street, Islington. It was here that there occurred a random incident which unexpectedly changed the direction of his life. The shop next door to his place of work was leased to a showman who exhibited freaks and novelties to the public. The initial amused contempt with which Tom Norman observed these activities was soon transformed into a thoughtful respect as he noted the steady stream of visitors who entered the shows each day. He joined the queue and paid a penny to see 'Mlle Electra', 'The Only Electric Lady – A Lady Born Full of Electricity'. He watched the sparks being drawn from various parts of her body and was startled to receive a distinct shock when he touched her hand.

It did not take much reflection to convince him that someone with his wits – 'a man with some capital and perhaps brains' was how he phrased it – might find a future in such a business. Within a few days he made the decision to finish with the meat trade for good and go into a business partnership with his neighbour. There was one disappointment in store: the discovery that 'Mlle Electra' was a fraud. She was connected to a lead from an induction coil, the other lead being attached to a metal plate that lay under a dampened carpet on which the customers stood as they viewed her.

Tom and his new-found partner set off with 'Mlle Electra' for Kingston Fair. According to the showman's patter, the 'Electric Lady' had been deaf and dumb since birth, but Tom soon discovered she 'had quite a lot to say, especially when it came to sharing up the takings'. She insisted on being allotted the lion's share and also regarded it as her right to sleep in a good class of apartment. The showman and his new assistant meanwhile passed their nights either in a tent or sleeping on boards under the barrow on top of which the show was stowed away. One night, lying underneath the barrow, Tom resolved that 'as soon as the bank was strong enough I must have a show of my own'. This he achieved with his own 'Electric Lady' in a shop in Hammersmith towards the end of the season. Takings were good, for he had learnt one basic lesson: more important than the exhibit were the techniques used to present it to the public.

But you could indeed exhibit anything in those days. Yes, anything from a needle to an anchor, a flea to an elephant, a bloater, you could exhibit as a whale. It was not the show, it was the tale that you told.

Panache and patter, the building up of the sense of expectation in casual listeners, drawing more of them in from among chance passers-by until you created your crowd – all of this counted for more than the material. He also made the discovery that he possessed an inherent talent for this style of showmanship and knew he had stumbled on his natural vocation.

Tom never divulged to any of his sons or daughters why he took the surname 'Norman', relinquishing that of Noakes along with his inheritance as the eldest son. There was a tradition among the descendants of his brother Charles that he changed his name on the insistence of the Noakeses since they found any association with 'circus folk' distasteful. Certainly it was nothing unusual in those days for a young man to change his name for the sake of family sensitivities when lured into abandoning a 'respectable' background for the vagabondage of circus or fairground life.

For a time Tom Norman's exhibitions travelled successfully from town to town, and his memoirs convey a vivid flavour of his tours. A suitable 'show shop' was the first requirement, preferably in the main street of the town being visited. Such premises were honestly hired as a rule, but if times were hard the use of a shop might be obtained by guile. The way it was done ran as follows. In mid-morning on a Saturday Tom Norman would approach an appropriate estate agent, stating he was acting for a new company that intended to open a chain of fancy bazaars. He would express interest in a vacant shop already earmarked and take the key, promising to return it on Monday morning. Since most estate agents had their own houses in the comfortable quiet suburbs, they never knew that no sooner did Tom Norman see them depart safely for home at about midday than he moved into the empty premises.

In no time the 'props' arrived on a small cart drawn by an old black man, who happened in this instance to be the show itself. A large canvas sheet, covered by an oil painting that bore at least a remote relationship to the entertainment about to be mounted, was then hung high up on the front of the building by a system of poles and pulleys. Tom Norman usually kept several such paintings in store, ready to be adapted to practically any class of freak. Whitening or soap was then used to write notices or 'gags' on the shop windows, sawdust was sprinkled on the floor and a large enamel Pears Soap advertisement sign was laid on the boards so that a coke fire could be lit in a bucket to heat the red-hot iron bars the old black man would later bite and bend.

During Tom Norman's earlier days, naphtha flares were used outside the show shops, but as these grew hot, the naphtha often began to drip on to the pavements and catch alight, becoming a hazard to passers-by. Later he adopted paraffin lamps, and when there was not enough money to buy oil for the six large lamps needed, the black man would be dispatched to the nearest stores to have 'three quarters of paraffin' put into each lamp. The man would tell the oilman that the lamps were now too heavy to carry all at once, so he would take three now and return for the others later. With the first three lamps the exhibition could be opened. As soon as enough money had been taken, the remaining three could be sent for and the bill settled.

When the exhibition was at last ready to take off, the black man, now clad in skins and feathers and with large curtain rings on his hands and legs and a ring in his nose, danced in the shop doorway, beating a gong or tom-tom. Tom Norman further enlivened the proceedings by telling tales of how this aged native once swam across the Orange River to save a party of shipwrecked sailors who would otherwise have been lost. (It was an element in the story he hastily discarded when a knowledgeable listener – such a person being termed a 'Noah's Ark' or 'nark' in showmen's lingo – informed him that anyone who wished to might wade across the Orange River without getting their knees wet.)

With Tom's 'touting, shouting and telling of the tale', it was seldom long before he had the thoroughfare completely blocked by people, and on occasion there could be trouble from an officious policeman. But such exhibitions were a common sight, and the police were usually readily persuaded to turn a blind eye while making a habit of looking in once during the evening, as a rule just before going off duty. Then Tom Norman, knowing what was expected, would slip the bobby sixpence for his trouble – always in coppers, since he thought it seemed a bigger sum in this form.

Throughout the Saturday afternoon and evening the show continued, often staying open till midnight. It opened for a while again on the Sunday, but by daybreak on Monday the props were safely packed on the cart and the show slipping quietly out of town. The key to the shop had been pushed through the estate agent's letter-box with a note of regret that the premises turned out to be unsuitable for the purpose in mind.

The shows Tom Norman exhibited changed frequently and he was willing to put on almost any display. The novelties he promoted included fleas in harness, fat ladies, giant babies, tall men, short men. For a 'Savage Zulu Show' he recruited his savages from among the ranks of retired seamen living in the lower depths of the Ratcliffe Highway. These painted themselves for the part, conversing before the customers in a gibberish of their own invention. Such shows were, of course, common enough on the fairgrounds, and it must have been one much like Tom Norman's that surely tested the patience of the citizens of Northampton, fed up with the frequent mounting of entertainments on their Market Square. On 4 June 1881, the *Northampton Mercury* recorded their complaint:

By permission of the Mayor, the proprietor of any show can pitch his tent on the Square at any time, and the latest example of the nuisance of which we are complaining occurred on Tuesday, when some Zulus were exhibited in a large booth. However estimable these gentlemen and ladies may be in other spheres, they have not proved themselves desirable neighbours in this case. During the evening they kept up a sort of exaggerated Gregorian chant, with Zulu variations, alternating with the strains of a powerful organ.

An Irish giant and an Irish dwarf, exhibited jointly as 'The Hibernian Contrarieties', made another striking attraction. Tom Norman also mounted the classic talking head illusion and, at a later date, even a 'wireless' demonstration, where the customers stood around the side of the room listening to music supposedly coming from London. In this case the moments of sharp disillusion were rather too frequent as the needle stuck on the gramophone in the back room.

One exhibition to which Tom Norman became particularly attached was his family of midgets. It consisted of two midgets, billed as man and wife and always brought into town in a specially constructed miniature coach drawn by ponies. In each town on the tour he made a point of closing the show down for a few days so as to allow the lady midget to 'give birth to her baby'. A new-born infant would then be hired to stand in for the hypothetical offspring, and even larger queues always gathered after such a 'happy event' to see the new arrival. The only problem was the difficulty he had in restraining the 'mother' from swearing volubly, smoking a pipe and drinking gin in front of the customers. The exhibition finally came to grief when the 'mother' ran away one night, objecting to being displayed as a woman any longer, both midgets being men.

But Tom Norman's ventures rarely ran utterly aground. He developed into a past master in the art of attracting the attention of a crowd with a versatility of stunts and tricks. One of his favourite gimmicks was to announce that a particular show was booked to appear at some future illustrious event – and at this point he usually invoked the name of P. T. Barnum, American proprietor of 'The Greatest Show on Earth'. It was a trick he tried once too often. One afternoon at Arcadia, held in the Royal Agricultural Hall, Islington, he boldly stated his usual claim, only to find he had set off unrestrained merriment on the part of three gentlemen in the audience. After the show, when he was introduced to them, one of them turned out to be no less a person than the great showman himself. Barnum stretched out a hand to touch the festoons of Mexican and American silver dollars that Tom Norman habitually wore suspended from his watchchain and said to his companions with wry amusement, 'The Silver King, eh?' – the phrase no doubt springing spontaneously to his lips as a reference to *The Silver King*, Henry Arthur Jones and Henry Herman's celebrated melodrama and stage hit of 1882. It was enough: from a moment of acute embarrassment Tom Norman characteristically salvaged triumph. He retained the nickname to the end of his days and claimed Barnum among his friends.

As his ventures prospered, so Tom found it possible to move into permanent premises. The first shop he took over was in the Edgware Road, but by the end of six months he was proprietor of thirteen more exhibition shops in and around London. He had a 'money-taker' at each and spent his time going from shop to shop to gather the takings, watch the progress of various displays, make minor adjustments to shows and move exhibits between premises.

He was now continually short of suitable novelties and freaks, and would go to immense pains to obtain new live showpieces, often making a long train journey on the strength of a friendly tip. Having come across a suitable subject for display, he would employ a skilful guile in his approach, perhaps spending several days at gaining the confidence of the person concerned before making a proposal. In speaking of the money his clients earned, he was apt to use phrases like 'star artist amounts' or 'princely salaries', and he claimed to have paid his living exhibits sums 'that enabled them to enjoy every reasonable luxury of life'.

Should anyone level at him the charge of exploiting his freaks for personal profit, he could defend himself by pointing out that his freaks were earning more than they could hope to by any other means. Besides, so long as they remained under his care they were no longer a burden on relatives or the community. He insisted that their lives as exhibition freaks were both varied and interesting, whereas the only real alternative was for them to be shut away in the dull seclusion of their homes or a workhouse. Nothing could have shaken his conviction that, for the most part, his freaks led happy and contented lives, or that he was offering them a positive alternative. While the Poor Law remained in force he had an unanswerable point.

It was during the early period when he was building up his small empire of exhibition shops in London that Tom Norman received the proposal from 'Little George' that he take on the London management of the grotesquely deformed young man from Leicester known as the Elephant Man. In due course, George Hitchcock and Joseph Merrick arrived in London one Thursday afternoon in November 1884. It was a day later than planned and Tom Norman was relieved to see them, though he had a 'second sight' act standing by to fill the bill at his Whitechapel shop the following week in the event of a vacancy in his plans. Meanwhile, in the East India Docks Road shop, he was promoting a contortion and acrobatics team known as the Dailo Sisters. They were to be replaced after the weekend by a Professor Durland with his 'Man Fish' and 'Transparent Lady' who were the current attraction at Whitechapel.

When Tom Norman first set eyes on Joseph Merrick, he saw him wearing not the startling get-up Treves describes, but, more conventionally, a long black coat, a black felt hat and a woollen muffler concealing the greater part of his face. Mr Hitchcock introduced the Elephant Man informally as 'Joe', a familiarity which at once jarred on Tom Norman's sensibilities. But his apprehensions deepened to dismay as Joseph removed his hat and coat and unwound his muffler. Though the showman considered himself to be accustomed to the strangest sights in nature, he had to confess that his unspoken response on first seeing Joseph was, 'Oh God! I can't use you.' Yet he was already committed by contract to the Midlands showmen, and besides, he detected a palpable depth of pleading and suffering in the Elephant Man's eyes.

'Well, Mr Meyrick, I'll call you Joseph if I may,' Tom Norman said, emphasizing the dignity of 'Joseph' over 'Joe' and shaking the Elephant Man by the hand. Privately he considered that if he had seen Joseph while he was still in the Leicester workhouse, he would never have been among the parties to his release. The shrewd suspicion was forming at the back of his mind that Sam Torr's group had all too quickly run into problems over displaying their client and were losing no time in passing him on. Nevertheless he noticed when George Hitchcock left to return to Leicester at the end of the day that the two men parted 'in a spirit of friendship'.

Tom Norman was quite used to living rough when the occasion demanded, though he was also adept at improvising modest comforts and was a stickler for cleanliness, insisting that his assistant Jimmy should sweep the shop out every morning. In the Whitechapel premises he had set up two 'small iron beds, one for myself and the other for any of my novelties who cared to use it'. There was also a large gas ring (the 'Bunsen burner' of Treves's recollection) that he surrounded with bricks to conserve the heat. It was effective, he claimed, both for keeping the room warm and for boiling a kettle.

With Joseph's arrival Jimmy was sent out to buy a new mattress and a couple of extra blankets for the bed. A curtain was also hung around the Elephant Man's bed area to give him at least a little privacy. Thus they had their 'rough and ready' comforts and Joseph seemed quite happy with the arrangements, the anxiety having meanwhile faded from his eyes. He referred in conversation to the workhouse, commenting that, 'I don't ever want to go back to that place.'

The Leicester consortium had sent down a set of 'rather crude posters depicting some monster half-man and half-elephant rampaging through the jungle'. Tom Norman saw these as more of a liability than a help, for Joseph was incapable of anything beyond a 'somewhat erratic walk'. But the posters were all they had to hang outside the shop and attract interest. There were also around one thousand copies of a freakshow pamphlet, to be sold at a halfpenny each, the proceeds constituting a contribution to Joseph's income.

By the time the show opened at midday on the Monday, Tom Norman had his walk-up patter worked out to explain the posters away as nothing more than attention-catching devices. 'The Elephant Man is not here to frighten you but to enlighten you,' he informed the lunchtime crowd, prudently adding that no lady in a 'delicate state of health' should enter the shop. As soon as he had gathered his audience and ushered them inside, he offered his introduction, shaped to a formula which could be adapted to every occasion and would hopefully forestall the comments of any smart alec or 'nark' who might be present:

> Ladies and gentlemen, in the absence of the lecturer, with your indulgence, I would like to introduce Mr Joseph Merrick, the Elephant Man. Before doing so I ask you please to prepare yourselves – Brace yourselves up to witness one who is probably the most remarkable human being ever to draw the breath of life.

As he next drew back the curtains to reveal Joseph on a low platform stage, he noted the gasp of horror that ran through the group of onlookers. Thus it was on each occasion. Neither was it unusual for one or more of the audience to depart hastily at this point in the proceedings as Tom Norman continued:

> Ladies and gentlemen, I ask you please not to despise or condemn this man on account of his unusual appearance. Remember we do not make ourselves, and were you to prick or cut Joseph he would bleed, and that bleed or blood would be red, the same as yours or mine.

The account of Joseph's mother being frightened by an elephant when she was in a 'delicate state of health' then followed in its place, with an explanation of how he had come to be in the Leicester workhouse until the chance of joining the showmen made his release possible, so enabling him to pay his way in the world, 'independent of charity'.

Tom Norman was adamant that at no time did he treat Joseph like a 'wild animal', as Treves implied. He pointed out that it would have been in neither his nature nor his interests to do so. It was his experience that a majority of the show's patrons responded with a degree of pity and sympathy after their initial shock. 'Had I attempted to be harsh with him . . . I would very soon have had the show wrecked, and me with it.'

One morning, a week or so after the Elephant Man's arrival in

London, Tom Norman awoke in the early hours and was startled to catch sight of Joseph through a gap in the curtains and to realize he was sitting up, his chin on his knees. When he asked if he was ill, Joseph replied that this was how he always slept. To lie down to sleep, he explained with a dark humour, would be to risk waking with a broken neck. Tom Norman wondered whether it might be possible to devise a form of support something like a milkmaid's yoke to ease Joseph's nights. He set his mind to work on the problem and called in Joe Wintle, a carpenter who often helped him out with odd jobs. Mr Wintle and his wife contrived a basketwork frame, padded with lambswool, that could be strapped to Joseph's shoulders and allow him to lie down. It was an ingenious attempt, but they were never able to make the contraption comfortable enough for it to function.

Business was satisfactory if not especially brisk. The pamphlet in particular was selling well. It would not be long before they needed to think about ordering fresh supplies. The steady stream of medical students and staff who had started to come across from the London Hospital to satisfy their curiosity was meanwhile turning into a mixed blessing. These visitors tended to stand about afterwards, asking questions, talking among themselves and holding up the next viewing. Tom Norman decided he must draw a firm line and insist that they clear the shop promptly. Shortly before the start of business one day, however, a young doctor approached and introduced himself as Dr Tuckett. His pleasant manner favourably impressed the showman, who agreed to the doctor's request to be allowed to meet the Elephant Man before the show opened. These three young men, each of them still aged less than twenty-five, then held a brief conversation that closed with Dr Tuckett asking if one of his colleagues, a Mr Treves, might be accorded the same privilege. Tom Norman unhesitatingly said yes.

His assistant Jimmy was a sharp twelve-year-old who would dress in a cast-off, brass-buttoned red waistcoat of his chief's to perform the most important of his duties: that of doorman. Jimmy had the responsibility of holding the door curtains closed and not letting anyone further in once a show was in progress. It had been impressed on him by his employer that his answer to any question about show, client or showman – whoever was doing the asking –

must always be, 'I don't know.' There was also a coded whistle, something like a donkey's 'hee-haw' reversed, that he was trained to use to signal trouble.

A morning or two after Dr Tuckett's overture Tom Norman was in Jack Winder's, a nearby coffee-shop, ordering breakfast for himself, Joseph and Jimmy. Their breakfasts consisted as a rule of a pair of kippers or bloaters, a jug of coffee, tea or cocoa, and a plate of 'doorsteps' of bread. While he waited he heard Jimmy's whistle and turned to see the boy pointing him out to a tall important-looking gentleman before doubling back to guard the shop. As Jimmy told the story later, Mr Treves 'didn't half want to know a lot, Guv'nor', but he had kept to his instructions and replied, 'I don't know,' to every question. In the end the exasperated Treves commented, 'You don't know much, do you?' To which Jimmy responded that he *did* know where Mr Norman could be found, but wouldn't tell for less than sixpence. Treves paid up and at last the showman and the eminent surgeon stood eye to eye.

It was a moment of mutual antipathy. Treves, thoroughly put out by the bother he had been through and awkward in the dingy surroundings, asked brusquely, 'Are you Norman, the showman?' 'That is my name, sir, unfortunately,' Tom Norman replied, the 'unfortunately' being a disarming little linguistic trick he used to break the ice with any new contact or acquaintance. It cut no ice with Mr Treves, and since it was obvious that he had no wish to tarry in Winder's coffee shop, Tom Norman suggested he wait outside till his order was completed. Once back at the show shop, Tom Norman treated Mr Treves to a quick run-through of the routine and patter, deciding he would allow him no more than a quarter of an hour. As soon as it was over he insisted that they must now get on with their breakfast.

Treves probably acted wisely when, later in the day, he sent the more tactful Reginald Tuckett back over the road to negotiate to bring the Elephant Man across to the hospital. Joseph himself raised no objection, while Tom Norman saw in the proposal both the advantage of publicity and the chance that Joseph might come by some medical advice. So far as he could remember in later years, there were in all two or three such visits to the London Hospital, but after the last of them Joseph dug in his heels and said he had no wish to go again. He did not mind, he said, being displayed discreetly and decently when he was being paid, but over there 'I was stripped naked, and felt like an animal in a cattle market'.

A further week passed before the next request was received, and this time Tom Norman turned it down. Frederick Treves arrived forthwith in some agitation, explaining how there were several distinguished visitors whom he had invited to meet Merrick. Tom Norman, perceiving that the surgeon was anxious over 'losing face among his colleagues', went in to Joseph to try to persuade him that he should perhaps go just one more time. But by now Joseph's obstinate streak was in the ascendant. He forthrightly refused. 'Treves could hardly control his rage,' wrote Tom Norman, 'at being told of Joseph's refusal, especially when I said that in future he and his colleagues could only see Joseph as paying customers.' Treves may have needed to hand the boy Jimmy sixpence for his trouble, but it seems there were none of the other financial arrangements he implied. For his part, to the end of his life, Tom Norman felt it was significant that, only a few days after this incident, the police moved to close the show.

The worst anyone could find to say about Tom Norman was that he had been a bit of a rascal in his youth – he admitted it himself. He could be disarming, even charming, in self-criticism, as when he remembered as an old man the 'very flash appearance' he once cultivated with his curly-brimmed bowler hat, his waistcoat jingling with watchchains and silver coins and his white gloves with ostentatious rings worn on the outside: 'always appearing to be up to the thousand pounds a year mark, and perhaps, if the truth were known, I did not possess a thousand pence ... I often think that my flashness proved to be a big asset.'

The contrast of the man as he showed himself to be with the surly, harsh image briefly conveyed by Frederick Treves in the opening passages of 'The Elephant Man' is striking. Treves claimed to have extracted Norman from a pub, but Norman describes a coffee-shop as their meeting ground and states he was a convinced teetotaller at that stage of his life. He was no fly-by-night nonentity, but a man who learned his trade inside out, lived intensely by his wits and founded a dynasty that continued to be active in fairground and circus circles for many years. He was known as one of the most enterprising of the English showmen, having been the second in the country, it was said, to introduce a steam generator to provide electric light on a fairground. In 1890 he also set up as a showman's auctioneer. In time he would act for such famous personalities as Lord George Sanger and the Bostock family, who had, of course, at an earlier stage, taken over the running of Wombwell's Menagerie.

Tom Norman felt he came to know Joseph Merrick well during the few weeks they were together. Of the reactions of the freakshop audiences he commented that, while 'they could not have admired his appearance, none could doubt his spirit'. Shortly before their paths divided he gained a further insight into Joseph's proud independence. With all the pamphlets sold and the new printing awaited, Joseph was temporarily deprived of this source of his income. A fellow showman suggested that they 'work the nobbings', which in showground slang meant passing round the hat for the performer's benefit. Yet Joseph would hear none of it. He turned at once to Tom Norman with the words, 'We are not beggars are we, Thomas?'

He also confided in the showman his dream of eventually having enough capital set aside to buy himself a small house where he might live quietly. The showman himself claimed that, if only Joseph had remained under his management, the dream could have been fulfilled. While this may be seen as wishful thinking after the event, the Silver King was also a man who might well have brought it off.

1. The portrait of Sir Frederick Treves by Luke Fildes that hangs in the London Hospital Medical College (*London Hospital*)

2. Dr Reginald Tuckett, who introduced Treves to the Elephant Man

3. The front of the London Hospital as it was in 1876, the new Grocers' Wing to the left of the main façade (*from* The Illustrated London News)

4. The earliest known illustrations of Joseph Merrick: the engravings from the
Transactions of the Pathological Society of London (1885)

5. Design from a broadsheet advertising Wombwell's Royal Menagerie

6–7. Engravings of Merrick's head, published in the *British Medical Journal* for
December 1886 but probably contemporaneous with Plate 4

8. The Leicester Union Workhouse in the 1850s, where Merrick was first admitted in 1879 (*Leicester Museums and Art Gallery*)

9. A surgical operation of the 1880s reflecting Merrick's experience in the Leicester Infirmary (*courtesy* The Practitioner)

10. The birth entry for Joseph Carey Merrick in the local Leicester register

11. The record of Joseph Merrick's discharge from the Leicester Union Workhouse (*Leicester Museums and Art Gallery*)

12. A hand-bill for Sam Torr's Gaiety Palace of Varieties, Leicester. It is possible that Joseph Merrick was first exhibited on its stage (left)

13. The back and front covers of the pamphlet containing Joseph Merrick's autobiography (*British Museum*)

14. The music-hall performer and entrepreneur Sam Torr dressed for his speciality number, 'On the Back of Daddy-O'

15. 'Professor' Sam Roper, travelling fair proprietor

16. Sam Roper's nephew, Bertram Dooley, dressed as one of 'Roper's Midgets' for the boxing booth

17. The 'pillar-box' cap and pelmet, devised by Sam Roper, on the cast of Merrick's head

18. Tom Norman, 'The Silver King'

19. The SS *Norwich* on which Merrick returned from his disastrous continental trip (*Great Eastern Railway Society*)

20–23. A set of four photographs of Joseph Merrick, showing his condition at the time of his admission to the London Hospital in 1886.

CHAPTER 7

A Travelling Life

When the police closed down the show shop in the Whitechapel Road, it could not be argued that they were acting in Joseph Merrick's best interests, but that was not what they had in mind. Whether or not it was Frederick Treves who laid a complaint against the exhibition, they were responding to a shift in public opinion that demanded a tightening up of the standards of what was considered fit for public viewing. The forces of respectability were making a determined onslaught. Reading between the lines of Tom Norman's account, it seems that the police action prompted the Leicester consortium to panic and withdraw the Elephant Man from his management.

Joseph, back on the road in the depths of winter, had gained little enough from his encounters with Frederick Treves and the Pathological Society of London. There had been no explanation offered for his illness, no hint of a possible treatment. The only souvenirs he evidently carried away were Treves's visiting card and a set of the photographs Treves had taken. One of the photographs was used as the basis for an illustration on the front of the new printing of the freakshop pamphlet, *The Autobiography of Joseph Carey Merrick*, that Tom Norman had been awaiting.

There is room for debate as to whether Joseph himself wrote the pamphlet or whether it was written for him. Those who read it must make their own judgement, but, on balance, the tone and content, the words and phrases, have a feeling of authenticity. Joseph was most likely its author, even if he did write it under the tutelage of Mr Torr or a resident copywriter. The fact that the birth date given is wrong may itself be seen as a confirmation of his authorship. As we know, he rarely got it right. In the illustration on the cover there is also a striking detail of artistic licence: the engraver has worked in the proto-'trunk', the extension of flesh that once protruded from the upper jaw but which the surgeons at the Leicester Infirmary had already removed.

Apart from the indignity of being a public exhibit, there is no reason to think that Joseph's life on the road was unremittingly harsh. Neither, despite Frederick Treves's views on the subject, was it lacking in friendship. The available evidence is quite to the contrary. Tom Norman's account amply demonstrates the protective instinct Joseph inspired among the showmen who handled his interests, and the principle seems to have held good for the next phase of his progress. Tom Norman stated that, to his certain knowledge, Joseph never saw the inside of a caravan up to the time he knew him, though he could not answer for what may have happened afterwards. It must therefore have been with the season of 1885 that Joseph's travels with Sam Roper's Fair began. According to a verbal tradition he was, during his time with the fair, allotted his own small caravan to journey in and so enjoyed a degree of privacy.

Two young men who worked in the boxing booth, billed as 'Roper's Midgets', befriended him at this time. These were Bertram Dooley and Harry Bramley, Bertram being a nephew of Sam Roper's by marriage and Harry his cousin. The present book is indebted to Bertram's son, Mr William Dooley, who was himself a professional illusionist on the variety stage under the stage name of Benson Dulay, for retelling his father's stories about the Elephant Man.

Bertram and Harry were in the habit of standing by to ward off any unwelcome attentions Joseph might attract. Bertram himself would make a point of visiting Joseph in his caravan to make sure all was well with him, and would sit and talk to him. He was, said Mr Dooley, impressed by Joseph's standard of conversation: 'A most interesting man – he would talk on subjects that you would never really think a man in that condition would talk about. Very upstage subjects, you know, and he was a bit on the religious side, too . . .' As for the outdoor garb and the theatrical cloak described by Frederick Treves: 'Uncle Sam thought of that, because the kids used to wait for him outside the fairground and follow him to the place where he slept.' Seemingly Tom Norman was therefore correct in his description of Joseph's mode of dress when he first arrived in London, and Frederick Treves, in another stroke of poetic licence, transposed the more dramatic get-up from a later occasion.

On one occasion with the fair set up on Market Square, Northampton, Joseph found himself being harassed by a group of town hooligans. Their ringleader took hold of the cloak to try to pull it away, but Harry came at once to the rescue, 'and laid the boy out, completely out. He must have hit him hard, but he was a good boxer, was Harry. He was a pretty broad, well-built chap, and he could use them . . .'

But the turn taken by events in Whitechapel Road, with the show closed down and moved on, had been a portent for the future. Sam Roper began to grow nervous about the way the Elephant Man drew the attention of local officialdom. The show was being kept under close scrutiny and Sam feared some sort of court case might be pending. The shocked reactions of the viewing public remained consistent. Possibly the idea was spreading that Joseph could represent a health hazard; that children especially ought not to be exposed to a risk of contact.

The main problem was that, as a freak, Joseph was almost too great a success. The showman's patter was designed to excite the imagination and anticipation of the crowd. Like the comedian's joke, it was the way it was told that counted. And the way it was told created a shared illusion with the audience that was all a part of acknowledged technique in the show business, as the old-timers referred to their profession. The trouble began when the audience actually set eyes on Joseph and the horror of his situation became all too immediate; and doubly disturbing for those sensitive enough to catch a glimpse of a living, suffering being inside the dreadful shell.

At the end of the freakshop pamphlet Joseph had quoted, or to be more exact misquoted, a verse from a poem by Isaac Watts (1674–1748), the English Nonconformist clergyman and poet who wrote some of the finest hymns in the Protestant heritage, two of the best-known being 'O God Our Help in Ages Past' and 'When I Survey the Wondrous Cross'. In its original form, in Watts's *Horae Lyricae*, Book Two, where it is part of a poem entitled 'False Greatness', the verse Joseph quoted runs as follows:

> Were I so tall to reach the pole,
> Or grasp the ocean with my span,
> I must be measured by my soul,
> The mind's the standard of the man.

The variations that Joseph introduces (see page 175; and also page 182) do nothing to alter the sentiment, and it may be that he was quoting from memory a verse that had stuck in his mind since childhood. Perhaps the words once appeared in his mother's Baptist hymnal. In the strange and pitiful case of the Elephant Man, Isaac Watts's words made their point well, though the old hymnographer could never have imagined the circumstances in which they now became so appropriate an assertion of human dignity. Nevertheless, those who felt affronted by the sight of Joseph made their complaints known.

The surgeon John Bland-Sutton had stated that: 'None would give him lodging except in an outhouse, or a stable, as if he were a wild animal.' It must have been true that his difficulty in keeping clean and the continual characteristic stench of his condition made him hardly an ideal touring companion. Yet, so far as the attitude of his managers went, Tom Norman was forthright in his protestations:

> I can honestly state as far as his comfort was concerned whilst with us, no parent could have studied their child more than any or all ... of us studied Joseph Meyrick's [sic] ...
> The big majority of showmen are in the habit of treating their novelties as human beings, and in a large number of cases, as one of their own, and not like beasts.

One of Tom Norman's boasts that he certainly made good was that the showmen acted in their exhibits' financial interests as much as in their own. The usual deal between showman and client was for an equal share of the takings. Whereas the showman then had to carry his overheads of rental, heating, lighting and other expenses, the client's share was clear profit. The client was moreover entitled to all the profits from the 'sellings', as souvenir pictures or pamphlets were termed. During the period of his exhibition, which Tom Norman stated was not above thirty months (it could, in fact, have only been twenty-two), Joseph accumulated savings of £50 from his share of the takings and the income from his pamphlet. At a time when whole families might have as little as £1 a week to subsist on, Joseph was able on the most conservative estimate to put aside between 10s. (50p) and 12s. (60p) a week. Fifty pounds was an appreciable nest-egg, sufficient to maintain him without working further and in reasonable comfort for a year at least and Tom Norman was to claim that he had considerably more than this set aside at the time when he left his care. Joseph was certainly quietly affluent, far better off than ever in his life, and better off than many who crowded the freakshows to view him.

But the difficulties were not dispersing with time. The opinion that freakshows were nothing more than exploitations of the afflicted for the entertainment of the ignorant continued to gain ground. Those with civic responsibilities saw it more and more as their duty to clamp down on all these and similar social evils wherever possible. Within the bounds of the City of London the tightening up was already achieved and the exhibition of monstrosities and freaks a feature of the past. Beyond the City's limits, in the sprawling inner suburbs, the display shops still flourished, for here authority lay in the hands of a diversity of overlapping parish and borough councils. With such a confusion of local governing bodies, no uniform policy was possible.

The East End, with its teeming working-class population, had long held special attractions for the showmen. There had always been freakshows in the East End, and the exhibitions of monstrosities and prodigies were, as we have seen, daily events in the Whitechapel and Mile End roads. Yet even here a sense of change was in the air, and few were more shrewdly aware of it than Tom Norman. It was proposed that the various London parishes and boroughs be amalgamated into a single giant authority, the London County Council. Within three years the Local Government Act of 1888 would make this union an accomplished fact. The newly formed authority would then spring into vigorous action, bringing social reform into every corner of the lives of the people. Within a matter of months all the freakshops would be swept away, and Tom Norman, his small empire in ruins, would find himself having to adopt fresh techniques on the showgrounds.

I well remember [he wrote] an old showman telling me of the change about to take place, and, 'Tom,' he added, 'when it does, your and my occupation is gone.' As far as the show shops are concerned, he was right. Those that do not believe me, just test it in one shop alone. Why you would get closed up, before you got open.

Already, in 1885, the cold draught was being felt in the freakshow business as police and magistrates became steadily more persistent in their opposition to the exhibition shops and the obstructions on pavements they tended to create. For the showmen, any exhibition that might attract both the attention and the opposition of the police was becoming less and less a desirable property. Fate had brought Joseph Merrick into his adopted profession a little too late.

We do not know exactly when the decision was taken to dispatch Joseph on a tour of the Continent. The thinking behind it was obvious: to avoid the increasing harassment of the English police and to go on show in countries where police and authorities might be expected to be more relaxed about such matters. It was also the case that the novelty value of the Elephant Man was wearing thin on the circuits available to Sam Torr, Sam Roper and the consortium.

One source states that the manager who took over Joseph Merrick's interests on the Continent was an Austrian. William Dooley, on the other hand, remembered his father saying that it had been an Italian 'with a name like Ferrari' who proposed the tour – 'an Italian born, but he was really the same as a cockney Italian, like the ice-cream version'. There was certainly a novelty showman called Joe Ferrari who was active in showground circles at this time, and who later worked in the United States, but whether he was the figure in the Elephant Man case is not proven. In Mr Dooley's words, 'Sam Roper got talking to him, and "Oh", he said, "I will put him in a show like yours, and I am going on the Continent", and he took the Elephant Man away from us, which Uncle Sam didn't mind really. He didn't want to lose him, but at the same time he felt there was something there for him, you know, and Ferrari took him away with him on to Belgium . . .'

Unfortunately for this showman and his new property, the police forces of Europe proved as resistant to the exhibition of Joseph's deformities as those in England. The tour was a failure from the start, leading Joseph ever closer to disaster. The police continually moved on and forbade the show, and after some months of shifting from place to place, it became clear to the manager that he had little hope of making any gain on the venture; that he had landed himself with a liability.

Some time in June 1886, the shadowy figure of Mr Ferrari finally abandoned the Elephant Man in Brussels, compounding his villainy by stealing all the money Joseph had managed to save. This was how Joseph came to awake one morning to find himself abandoned and destitute in a foreign city where he had neither friends nor hope of assistance, and where he was quite unable to communicate with those about him. For any normal person it would have been unpleasant enough, but for Joseph it was catastrophic. His predicament was extreme, and his one thought can have been to somehow get back to England. With difficulty he pawned the few possessions he was left with, raising barely enough to pay for his passage home.

Frederick Treves's account is far too condensed to help with disentangling the course that events now followed.

> The impresario, having robbed Merrick of his paltry savings, gave him a ticket to London, saw him into the train and no doubt in parting condemned him to perdition.
> His destination was Liverpool Street.

The point is already made that savings of £50 were far from paltry by the standards of ordinary working people, and Joseph's journey to his home country was nothing like the relative plain sailing that Treves implies. In 1886 the established cross-channel route from Brussels to England was by way of Ostend and Dover, the Hook of Holland terminal familiar to modern travellers not being established until 1893. There was an alternative route to Harwich, and thence to Liverpool Street, but this went round by way of Rotterdam, a long way to the north and a longer and more expensive journey. A through ticket from Brussels to Liverpool Street is therefore unlikely. It makes more sense to see Joseph making his way to Ostend in the hope of catching the regular packet service for Dover, which would in due course have delivered him into London at Victoria Station.

And it is at Ostend that we next have news of him, though the saga of his journey home was already entering its most wretched phase as he travelled on the train from Brussels. To his own consciousness inside his poor distorted skull, in an advancing state of bewilderment and panic, it must have seemed that he was on the road to his final crucifixion. The faces of strangers who spoke in languages he could not understand pressed against the carriage windows and gaped in attempts to catch a look beneath the great hat's veilings. If he descended from the train, the crowd mercilessly followed after his bizarre shuffling figure whichever way it tried to turn. At Ostend a blow as savage as any fell when the captain of the cross-channel ferry, appalled by Joseph's appearance and mindful of the feelings of his other passengers, refused to allow him aboard.

That he turned out to be not entirely friendless in Ostend even in these circumstances was a piece of fortune he certainly deserved. 'I have had the most awful case in my care at Ostend,' wrote Wardell Cardew to the well-known actor of the day, W. H. Kendal, referring to the Elephant Man. Mr Cardew, it seems was someone with medical connections who was able to offer Joseph the help and shelter he so desperately needed at that point. Perhaps it was on his advice that Joseph next made his way back north along the coast for sixty miles to the Belgian port of Antwerp. From Antwerp the regular packet service to Harwich was well established. It had been in operation since 1864 and worked as a branch of the Great Eastern Railway.

By 1886 the service was daily except Sundays, the run being shared by three 'railway' steamers. The senior ship of the team was the paddle steamer *Princess of Wales*, built in 1878 and joined in 1883 by a pair of ships, the S.S. *Norwich* and the S.S. *Ipswich*. These were the first Great Eastern Railway packet ships to be propelled by twin screws rather than paddles. It was, in fact, the S.S. *Norwich* that made the crossing on the night of 23 June and so delivered Joseph back to the shores of his homeland.

The second-class fare from Antwerp to London was 15s. (75p) at this time, and must have taken the last remnant of Joseph's money. At least he succeeded in passing muster at the gangplank and getting himself aboard. The departure time from Antwerp was at 17.00 hours, so the long 150-mile crossing of the North Sea took place mostly during the hours of darkness. Joseph doubtless spent the night passage suffering from cold and hunger out on the decks, seeking a spot where he might merge into the shadows and be sheltered from the wind as well as the eyes of fellow passengers.

Docking time at Harwich was shortly after 4 a.m. As he shuffled wearily along the boat train in the disorientating light of early dawn, searching for a carriage where he might sit in isolation, Joseph perhaps felt a momentary sense of relief at regaining the relative sanctuary of his own country. At 5 a.m. the final stage of his journey began as the train pulled out of Harwich to carry him over the last sixty-five miles to London. Its scheduled time of arrival at Liverpool Street was ten minutes to seven.

Did Joseph sleep away the journey, or were his thoughts coherent enough for him to turn over the problems now facing him? These were surely immense, and to all appearances insoluble.

For several days he had been travelling towards a destination that did not really exist beyond the ending of the tracks at Liverpool Street Station. His resources were expended, his energy exhausted. What the next step should be was a question that found no answer. Circumstances had deprived him of the last remote hope he had of paying his way in the world; his only security, his savings, had been stolen. Liverpool Street was a metaphorical as well as a physical terminus and Joseph Merrick's destiny was finally and utterly taken out of his own hands.

It is unlikely that Sam Torr, Tom Norman or Sam Roper could have been of much help to him by this stage. His value as a novelty had worn thin and the moral opposition was formidable. In any case, Mr Torr had his own problems. The response in Leicester to the 'quality' music-hall fare with which he attempted to provide the town had proved disappointing. The Gaiety at the Gladstone Vaults was closed by now, pending new management, and Mr Torr was back in London, picking up the threads of his career as a *lion comique* on the halls.

Strangers who were approached by Joseph recoiled in horror

and revulsion and made no attempt to understand the broken speech from his lips. There was no hotel or lodging house that would receive him; no café or restaurant that would serve him; no hospital that would accept him as a patient, for he could neither share a public ward nor pay for a private one, and his condition was obviously incurable and untreatable. Only at a workhouse might he demand admission, and even there he would be eligible as a transient vagrant for no more than one night's stay. The next morning he would be obliged to pay for his lodging by labour in the work sheds before being turned out to walk the thirty miles or so to the next workhouse or 'spike', for vagrants were never allowed to stay two consecutive nights in any Poor Law institution unless it was the one serving the parish in which they were accepted as resident. Only at Leicester would the Board of Guardians seriously consider letting him become a permanent charge on the rates. And Leicester lay ninety-eight miles from London, even supposing he could summon the strength to walk such a distance; and in the knowledge that once the doors of that terrible place next closed again behind him it must be for ever.

When Joseph Merrick finally arrived on the platforms of Liverpool Street Station amid the steam, smoke and bustle of a Victorian railway terminus awakening into life in the early morning of 24 June 1886, it was as it always had been for him, yet even worse. His will was gone, his demoralization complete. The attention his figure drew was instant, whether he tried to move on or stood stock-still. The crowd gathered with its murmuring comments, the fingers pointed, the eyes stared. Early travellers paused, wondering at the cause of the commotion, and the crowd grew, acting as a magnet for newcomers who pressed ever closer in their attempts to obtain a glimpse.

It was the police who stepped in and forced back the by now highly excitable crowd, guided the helpless, terrified and extraordinarily top-heavy little figure into the haven of the third-class waiting-room; then held the doors against the press of people who clamoured to be allowed a sight of the strange being that had come among them. Freed from the buffetings of the human storm outside, Joseph collapsed into the furthest and darkest corner of the room. The policemen who leaned over the evil-smelling, huddled bundle could make nothing of the high-pitched, run-together words it tried to utter. They saw only that with one evidently uncrippled hand it fumbled in an interior pocket and brought out and offered a small oblong of much-thumbed pasteboard.

The police inspected the card. It had on it the name of a gentleman apparently connected with the London Hospital. They knew the London Hospital well enough. It was a little over a mile away and the place to which every victim of an attempted suicide or murder, every unfortunate injured in a street accident or fight, would be referred on that side of London. The gentleman should be sent for to see what advice he could offer or what light he could throw on this odd, disturbing traveller.

Frederick Treves's day's work at the hospital can hardly have begun on that morning of 24 June 1886 when the message arrived asking him to go to assist the police at Liverpool Street Station. When he arrived the crowd about the waiting-room was still so thick that the surgeon had some trouble in pushing his way through. As at length he managed to get in at the door and to enter the waiting-room, the figure of the Elephant Man immediately rang a bell of recognition. It was huddled close against the wall as if trying to shrink away to nothing. Treves realized that the man must by now be beyond the limits of endurance and utterly broken.

After a few words with the police, the surgeon agreed to take responsibility. With their help he shepherded or half-carried the staggering Joseph out through a crowd to where a hansom cab waited. They bundled him in, and instructions were given to the driver as Treves himself clambered into the confined interior. The Elephant Man questioned nothing, but sat in a silent daze, seemingly all at once overcome with a great, trusting sense of calm. Then, as the cab turned out of the station, he sagged into a sudden and astonishingly childlike sleep.

As they clattered through the streets, Treves, sitting in the cab filled with the well-remembered stench of Joseph's body, must have begun to consider the implications of the responsibility he had accepted. The righteous system by which society sought to control the lives of the poor and destitute could offer Joseph nothing to meet his true needs. At best they might shut him away in the anonymous harshness and squalor of an institution to await his death and so erase himself from the world's consciousness. The rules themselves were founded on the Protestant ethic at its most perverse: that material prosperity represented the natural reward of virtue. Joseph and those like him had no business to exist.

Frederick Treves's mind was made up that the time had come for the rules to be broken, and he was prepared to use his own prestige to that end. Having descended in his hansom cab like a *deus ex machina* to rescue a broken life, he intended to see the role through. If his last approach to Joseph had been met by rebuff, he laid the blame for that firmly on the shoulders of the showman Tom Norman.

The hansom cab, with its incongruous pair of passengers, returned to the London Hospital, where Joseph was helped to a small, single-bedded isolation ward tucked away up in the attics. Here he was washed, given food, put to bed, and for the moment left to sleep and dream.

There was only one brief disruption to his new-found peace and quiet when a nurse bringing food, and not forewarned of what to expect, came through the doorway and saw the figure of Joseph for the first time. The tray she was carrying crashed with its contents to the floor as the woman screamed and ran off down the corridor. But Joseph, propped up exhausted against his pillows, seemed too weak to notice the commotion.

CHAPTER 8

Come Safely into Harbour

A little short of six months after Joseph Merrick's unorthodox not to say positively irregular admission to the London Hospital, readers of *The Times* opened their copies on Saturday, 4 December 1886, to find a letter that was attention-catching even within the individualist tradition of that newspaper's correspondence column. It was written by Mr F. C. Carr Gomm, chairman of the London Hospital management committee, and in effect launched an appeal, not on behalf of any fund for medical relief or general charitable cause, but for an individual. The uniqueness of the circumstances needed to be well defined for such an appeal to be justified. It began:

Sir,

I am authorized to ask your powerful assistance in bringing to the notice of the public the following most exceptional case. There is now in a little room off one of our attic wards a man named Joseph Merrick, aged about twenty-seven, a native of Leicester, so dreadful a sight that he is unable even to come out by daylight to the garden. He has been called 'the elephant man' on account of his terrible deformity. I will not shock your readers with any detailed description of his infirmities, but only one arm is available for work.

In the paragraphs that followed, Carr Gomm outlined the Elephant Man's history: how, some time before, Mr Treves, one of the hospital surgeons, saw him on exhibition. How the police stopped the exhibition and Merrick went to Belgium under the care of 'an Austrian manager' who left him robbed and destitute. How he pawned his last possessions, which raised his fare to England, where he felt that 'the only friend that he had in the world was Mr Treves of The London Hospital'. How the crowd had made his journey home an utter nightmare, and how when he arrived at the hospital he had 'only the clothes in which he stood'.

He has been taken in by our hospital, though there is, unfortunately, no hope of his cure, and the question now arises what is to be done with him in the future.

He has the greatest horror of the workhouse, nor is it possible, indeed, to send him to any place where he could not insure privacy, since his appearance is such that all shrink from him.

The Royal Hospital for Incurables and the British Home for Incurables both decline to take him in, even if sufficient funds were forthcoming to pay for him.

Mr Carr Gomm then reviewed in detail the administrative difficulties Joseph's case had raised, but made the point that, as an incurable, he ought not to be taking up space in an already overcrowded general hospital, 'where he is occupying a private ward, and being treated with the greatest kindness – he says he has never before known in his life what quiet and rest were'. Joseph's appearance, said Carr Gomm, was so terrible that

... women and nervous persons fly in terror from the sight of him, and that he is debarred from seeking to earn his livelihood in any ordinary way, yet he is superior in intelligence, can read and write, is quiet, gentle, not to say even refined in his mind. He occupies his time in the hospital by making with his own available hand little cardboard models, which he sends to the matron, doctor, and those who have been kind to him. Through all the miserable vicissitudes of his life he has carried about a painting of his mother to show that she was a decent and presentable person, and as a memorial of the only one who was kind to him in life until he came under the care of the nursing staff of The London Hospital and the surgeon who has befriended him.

It is a case of singular affliction brought about through no fault of himself; he can but hope for quiet and privacy during a life that Mr Treves assures me is not likely to be long.

It was symptomatic of the spirit of the times that Carr Gomm found it necessary to emphasize not only that Joseph was in no position to do an honest day's work, but also that no moral taint attached to his plight. To be utterly deserving of charity it was essential to be utterly virtuous. Oddly and evidently, Joseph's character did approximate to such an ideal, and many of those who met and came to know him would have agreed without question. The fact perhaps made Carr Gomm's task of raising the appeal easier, and he threw open an invitation to the influential readers of *The Times* to put forward suggestions for Joseph's future. He also made it clear that there was no question of the hospital ejecting the patient on to the street, even though it was at this stage in its history having to deal with some 76,000 cases a year.

I have never before been authorized to invite public attention to any particular case, so it may well be believed that this case is exceptional.

Any communication about this should be addressed either to myself or to the secretary at The London Hospital.

As it happened, a complex series of perplexities and discussions had led to the drafting of Carr Gomm's remarkable letter. Frederick Treves had deposited an administrative dilemma on the laps of the hospital committee when he acted to commandeer the small room tucked away among the attics in the roof of the East Wing. It was one among a set of rooms that had been converted to accommodate single private patients or isolation cases suffering from highly infectious diseases. The very act of admission was in technical breach of hospital regulations, as Treves himself recollected.

Chronic cases were not accepted, but only those requiring active treatment. I applied to the sympathetic chairman of the committee, Mr Carr Gomm, who not only was good enough to approve my action but who agreed with me that Merrick must not again be turned out into the world.

For the time being, it had been a question of ignoring the

irregularities of Joseph's presence in the hospital, and Treves had been free to examine Joseph at leisure. He was startled at the deterioration in physical health that had taken place during the past year and a half. The Elephant Man presented a pitiful sight: his deformities had increased to the point where their crippling effects were becoming more general; he had also developed bronchitis, and there was at least the suggestion of a heart disorder in an early stage. Eighteen months before, at the meeting of the Pathological Society of London, Treves had been able to note how Joseph enjoyed good health, how he was free from other serious disease apart from his condition, how he even possessed a fair degree of natural strength. Now he was driven to recognize that Joseph's expectancy of life could be no more than a few more years at the most.

After his admission to the London Hospital, Joseph's general condition remained poor for several days. Gradually a combination of food and rest helped him to recover some of his lost strength. The problem of the stink that arose from his skin was resolved more easily than might have been expected, for it was found that so long as he bathed once or twice a day, the odour could be reduced to a level which was hardly noticeable. It was also arranged that he should be attended only by nurses who volunteered, and that each of these be carefully prepared for his appearance before being admitted to the room. In this way the usual shocked reactions of people seeing him for the first time were avoided.

He remained, even so, a difficult patient to nurse. His speech was almost incomprehensible and he showed suspicion towards anyone who approached him. It was becoming clear that his spirit had suffered even more than his body from his recent experiences. Every knock on the door of the room, Treves noticed, provoked a reaction of startled anxiety. He flinched from the hands of his nurses, and he shook with agitation whenever a stranger entered his room or some thoughtless, sensation-seeking wardmaid or porter pushed the door of the room ajar to take a peep through the crack.

For many days Joseph remained unsettled and apprehensive, but at last the steady routine of hospital life and a growing familiarity with the doctors and nurses soothed his shattered nerves. He settled into a cautious watchful repose. He began to form tentative friendships with the hospital staff, expressing a shy but deep gratitude for everything they did for him. His manner, always gentle, now became almost serene, and he developed a childlike faith in those who tended him. The nurses would bring him cardboard cutouts from the toy shop to help him pass the time, and together they struggled to construct the models. Each finished model would then be solemnly presented to some member of staff as a token of the gratitude he felt but for which he could never find sufficient expression in words.

As time went on, Treves grew increasingly accustomed to the Elephant Man's odd speech and found he was able to talk with him and study him more easily. There were fresh examinations to be made and measurements to be taken; again Joseph was persuaded to strip and pose for the clinical photographer. At least there was for Treves, as he visited Joseph each day, the professional satisfaction of seeing a slow return to relative health. But simultaneously there hung between them – unspoken, even evaded – the matter of Joseph's future.

By November 1886, the blind eye of the authorities could not remain turned for much longer. Five months had gone by since Joseph's admission, and while he could still hardly be described as fit, it was obvious that little further improvement could be expected from the treatment the hospital had to offer. He was, moreover, occupying a private ward, urgently needed for other patients and for which no payment was being received. There were no other institutions that could be persuaded to offer him shelter, and even the hospitals for the chronic sick approached by Carr Gomm refused to give him a place. It seemed unthinkable that he should be callously discharged into the street, yet no funds were available to maintain him in a hospital ward where, by all the rules, he was an inadmissible case. Carr Gomm felt he could go no further without the authority of the full house committee.

At this point in the history of the Elephant Man a vigorous publicity campaign was set in motion on his behalf, though by whom it was originated is unclear. The fact is that events moved fast, the starting point having been a strikingly apposite sermon preached by the Master of the Temple, Dr Charles John Vaughan, on Advent Sunday, 28 November 1886. Dr Vaughan had achieved his present eminence only by living down a homosexual love affair with a pupil that had, in 1859, compromised and put an end to his career as a headmaster of Harrow School.

For his Advent sermon he took his text from the Gospel According to St John: 'Who did sin, this man or his parents, that he was born blind?' Was his choice of text coincidence, or did he speak from a knowledge of Joseph's distress? In theory his attention could have been drawn to the case of the Elephant Man by Carr Gomm, who was himself a barrister of the Inner Temple. If this was so, Dr Vaughan might have been expected to take a personal interest, for he also was born and spent his childhood years in the city of Leicester, where his father was vicar of the parish church of St Martin's.

Dr Vaughan's sermon in turn gave Carr Gomm the chance to cite it when, two days later, he took up his pen to write to *The Times*. By preaching eloquently on the text concerned, said Carr Gomm, Dr Vaughan had shown how 'one of the Creator's objects in permitting men to be born to a life of hopeless and miserable disability was that the works of God should be manifested in evoking the sympathy and kindly aid of those on whom such a heavy cross is not laid'. The letter was accordingly printed on the Saturday, and three days afterwards, on Tuesday, 7 December, the house committee made the whole problem of Joseph Merrick's future care the first item on the agenda to its routine weekly meeting.

As the committee minutes concisely record, Mr Carr Gomm began, as chairman, by addressing the meeting on Joseph's behalf, outlining the steps already taken and reviewing the background to the case as well as the circumstances that had led to the appeal in *The Times*.

The Chairman stated that the result had been the receipt of a very large number of letters and a considerable sum of money. About £100 had been sent for his help and a Mr Singer had offered to contribute £50 yearly if Merrick were kept here. (The only other suggestions the Chairman had received were to send him to a Hospital for the Blind, to Lighthouses or to Dartmoor.)

The House Committee considered this case very carefully and it was resolved to keep J. Merrick here for the present and the Chairman said that he would communicate with Mr Singer who made his liberal offer on Merrick's behalf.

The outcome was a public response that was literally astounding. Letters continued to arrive by every post. Even the *British Medical Journal* was moved on the following Saturday, 11 December, to investigate the incident with a mixture of aroused curiosity and professional detachment:

A letter from Mr Carr Gomm, Chairman of The London Hospital, appeared last week in *The Times*. It contained an appeal to the charitable public on behalf of John [*sic*] Merrick, a man afflicted by so terrible a deformity that he cannot venture out by daylight to the garden of the hospital. Not only does his condition prevent him from being kept in a public ward or admitted into an institution for incurables, but he cannot travel even by public conveyances. Among the other experiences of this kind, acutely painful to his feelings, a steamboat captain refused on one occasion to take him as a passenger.

The journal went on to dispose of any idea that Merrick suffered from elephantiasis, and reminded its readers that he had already featured in notices of the meetings of the Pathological Society of London, the case being then fully reported in the society's *Transactions*, when a plate was also featured.

Since that plate was taken the disease has made great progress. Through the kindness of Mr Treves, we have been supplied with four photographs, representing the patient's present condition. A comparison of these drawings with the plate above noted will show how the disease has advanced during the past two years . . .

We learn from Mr Treves that he has received piles of correspondence from the curious and from the charitable on the subject; and we trust that poor John Merrick will, through the efforts of the benevolent, be enabled to end his days in peace and privacy, with a small competence.

The report in closing rounded off with a rather technical discussion of Joseph's deformities, and there can be little doubt that it was inspired by Treves himself. Not only did it acknowledge his help, but it also contained the curious mistake that was the hallmark of all his writings on the topic of the Elephant Man: the erroneous statement that his Christian name was John. Whereas the hospital authorities, Carr Gomm and the editor of *The Times* managed without trouble to record him correctly as Joseph, Treves invariably and persistently referred to him as John Merrick.

So far as the disposal of Joseph's future was concerned, however, the situation was beginning to grow clearer by the next appointed meeting of the hospital committee on Tuesday, 14 December; was, indeed, happily resolving itself. The reverberations from the letter in *The Times* stirred up responses in many other newspapers, and these in turn took up the story. The plight of the Elephant Man was even carried in the provincial press, and reached, it seems, the hairdresser's saloon in the back streets of Leicester where Joseph's uncle Charles Merrick pursued his modest, hardworking trade. A 'very great number of letters had been received about Joseph Merrick', Carr Gomm was able to tell the hospital committee,

... and a very large sum of money upwards of £230 had been sent to him. No useful suggestion had been made for the best means of providing for the unfortunate man, save that his uncle had offered to take him in, but it appeared that there was an obstacle to this in the necessity Merrick was under of frequent bathing. Thus a considerable sum of money had been received, and as one gentleman, Mr Singer, had given £50 which he proposed to continue annually, it was the Chairman's opinion that the best course to pursue was to keep Merrick here. This course was agreeable to Merrick himself, and although he was not strictly admissible it seemed that it was the right thing to keep him here.

In this opinion the Committee unanimously agreed and the Chairman undertook to write to *The Times* announcing that his letter had been adequately answered.

It would be impossible to grudge Joseph his luck at last in the destiny that had besieged his life from its beginning. He had all at once caught the imagination of the British public in a way that could never have been possible while he remained a grotesque, disturbing showpiece in the freakshops. Only six months before it had seemed impossible to visualize any future for him beyond the inevitability of his being drawn down into Victorian England's insatiable and nameless maw for the destitute and broken in spirit. He also had the advantage of being the perfect object for philanthropic attention: utterly blameless, hence unqualifiedly deserving.

He had entered into his refuge.

Once it was all settled that Joseph remain resident in the London Hospital, it was essential for suitable living accommodation to be set aside and prepared. At the back of the hospital, between the high buildings of the East Wing and the new Grocers' Wing (so called because its building had been made possible by a generous donation from the Grocers' Company of the City of London), lay the sunny, echoing courtyard known colloquially as 'Bedstead Square'. It was christened thus because it was here that the iron bedsteads from the hospital wards were brought for repair, cleaning and repainting. On one side of the square, a flight of concrete steps led downwards from the courtyard to a small wooden door with a grimy overhead fanlight. Behind the door, bare and unused in the basements of the East Wing, were two small rooms. It was decided that these could make an ideal conversion into the Elephant Man's future home.

The task of overseeing the adapting of the rooms fell to Mr William Taylor, chief engineer to the hospital. He was in his early fifties, having come there in 1878 as an employee of the engineering firm which installed the lifts. Once the contract was completed, he was invited to stay on as a member of the hospital's engineering team and to help ensure that the lifts continued to work satisfactorily. Gradually he rose in rank to chief engineer, acquiring with his post the resonant title of 'Mechanical Engineer in Charge of the Artisan Staff'.

As a consequence of Mr Taylor's labours, the larger, outer room in Bedstead Square was furnished as a bed-sitting room. It had in it a table and chairs, a small fireplace with its own mantelpiece and a pleasant specially built armchair. The bed, too, had been specially constructed by the hospital works department. It still survived, tucked away in a storeroom, as late as the 1930s, an eyewitness describing it as a couch type of bed, 'carved or eased to accept his abnormal frame', covered in leather, probably over horsehair, and very hard to sit on.

The room gathered daylight from glass panels set within the door, from the fanlight above and from a narrow, deep-set sash window that looked on to the alley and the flight of concrete steps. On the inner wall of the room another door opened into a passageway, beyond which lay the second, smaller room of the suite. Here Mr Taylor managed to contrive a bathroom for Joseph's use. There were no mirrors in either room; this was the one firm stipulation that Frederick Treves laid down in the matter of furnishing.

The removal of Joseph to his new quarters was easily accomplished, but convincing him that the rooms were truly his for as long as he needed them turned out to be more difficult. It was all so much more than he had or could have hoped for. At a stroke he was provided with the sanctuary he had sought ever since the first time he ran away from home. The small basement rooms brought him a degree of privacy beyond his dreams. Their very remoteness from the general life of the hospital gave him security.

He surveyed them with an air of wonder, but his good fortune was too bountiful for him to be able to grasp all at once. He could only accept it with bewildered surprise and a barely comprehending gratitude. Meanwhile, with Joseph finally settled in quarters of his own, Treves in no way relinquished his care of his patient. He made a point of visiting him each day, and instructed his house surgeons to follow his example.

The position of house surgeon was a six-monthly appointment, and the honour of acting in this capacity was much sought after by newly qualified doctors, despite the fact that it was an unpaid labour, involving many long hours of work in the general wards, receiving room and operating theatre. Among these many chores, the visit to Joseph was not always regarded as the most welcome of routine tasks.

One of the first of the young doctors to find himself undertaking the duty was Wilfred Grenfell, a student of Treves who eventually achieved fame as Sir Wilfred Grenfell of Newfoundland, where he worked as a doctor attached to the Christian missions among the great fishing fleets of those days. In his autobiography, *A Labrador Doctor*, he wrote of the period when the Elephant Man came under his care, recording how Joseph was exceedingly sensitive about his appearance, yet pathetically proud of his normal left arm. He felt that in spite of everything, Joseph managed to keep up a cheerful disposition, and described how he would speak freely as he speculated on how he would look preserved in 'a huge bottle of alcohol – an end to which in his imagination he was fated to come'.

Grenfell attempted to measure the Elephant Man's hat, but found that his arms could not reach about its circumference. He also recorded how, in due course, the accommodation in Bedstead Square came to be called 'the Elephant House'. 'Only at night could the man venture out of doors, and it was no unusual thing in the dusk of nightfall to meet him walking up and down in the little courtyard.'

Dr Tuckett, who was responsible for Treves's initial visit to the Elephant Man, similarly remembered from his tour of duty the intense pride that Merrick took in his good arm. He too spoke of his love of beauty, his great gentleness of character and the fascination fine clothes held for him. He thought also that he would probably have been quite a good-looking young man if he had not suffered from such a frightful disability.

Someone who found that visiting the Elephant Man had more to it of duty than pleasure was Dr D. G. Halsted, who held the appointment in 1887 and whose own book of memoirs, *A Doctor in the Nineties*, was published as late as 1959. He seems to have found that Joseph had a consistently dispiriting effect on his own state of mind. In the patient's features he could make out nothing of the suggested resemblance to an elephant; rather he felt that the deformed face was more like that of a tapir, 'but I suppose a "Tapir Man" would not have been such a powerful attraction as a sideshow'. He could never bring himself to see Joseph as anything but pathetic, yet he would try to cheer him up if he found him miserable and depressed. He confessed that he always felt happier when, duty done, he could slip away to other responsibilities.

While Treves continued to pay at least one visit a day to the basement rooms, it also became his habit to spend a couple of hours in Joseph's company each Sunday morning. He deliberately set out to study and cultivate an understanding of his patient, and grew fluent in interpreting the distorted speech from Joseph's lips. It was therefore inevitable that he should become the person most closely acquainted with the Elephant Man. On Joseph's side, the pleasures of educated conversation were a new experience that he seized on eagerly. It was as though there existed in him a passion for talking that had lain dormant for lack of comprehending company. Now his Sunday mornings would pass in a pleasant haze of chatter with Treves.

At the time when he had carried out his first clinical examination two years earlier, Treves's assumption was that Merrick was more or less imbecilic. It was an impression reinforced by the trouble Joseph had in giving outward sign to inner feelings. His facial deformities prevented him from forming any expression, either of pleasure or grief, and the movements of his limbs were so clumsy that any gesture had lost all spontaneity by the time it reached completion. Only by a use of words was he able to convey his thoughts, and since his speech was as distorted as his mouth, his genuine intelligence and awareness could tend to go unrecognized.

In the early days of their conversations, Treves tried to manoeuvre Joseph into talking about his past, but here he encountered many gaps and odd reticences. ('It was a nightmare, the shudder of which was still upon him.') There were undoubtedly areas of trauma in Joseph's remembrance of his early life, and walls of silence that Treves never succeeded in breaching, despite their special relationship. While Joseph was willing to acknowledge he came from Leicester, he would never talk of his childhood there. He gave Treves the impression that he knew nothing whatsoever of his father; never did he mention his crippled sister, Marion Eliza, nor his dead little brother, William Arthur. Of his mother he did speak a little, but his description of her was so surrounded by a romantic and idealized glow that Treves firmly believed it to be only an elaboration of Joseph's deeply wounded imagination. Treves's insight was probably correct in so far as Joseph had eliminated from his memory the fact of her, too, being a cripple.

Joseph would talk of his mother as beautiful, and his most precious possession remained the small painted portrait of her that he carried everywhere and had managed to preserve through many vicissitudes. When Carr Gomm was first shown the picture, he sensed how Joseph displayed it with pride. It was as though the picture served as a constant reassurance that while Joseph was himself so hideously disfigured, at least he could preserve a myth of coming from undisfigured stock.

The perplexity Joseph felt in the matter of his own distorted body was once expressed to Treves in a remark he made about how odd it was that he should be so deformed when his mother had been so beautiful. He could never speak of her without his emotions welling over, and he never told Treves she was dead. It was this that led the surgeon privately to conclude that Joseph's mother abandoned him when he was still an infant. In fact all Joseph's memories of Mary Jane Merrick were those of a mother who had shown her son a constant gentleness and unfailing love.

If he could not be persuaded to talk of his family, neither would he discuss his experiences as an exhibit in the freakshows. He did, however, constantly perplex Treves by refusing to disparage the showmen who had managed him, stressing only the gratitude he felt towards them. By contrast, his memories of the workhouse invariably caused an outburst of bitter indignation. It was clear that returning to such an institution was intolerable for him to contemplate. Yet in all other things he gave the impression of looking back on his life without rancour and of accepting his misfortunes with quiet resignation. If there was bitterness at the indignities to which fate had submitted his physical body, he gave no sign.

Treves, as he listened, found himself increasingly fascinated by the world Joseph seemed to inhabit. The ideas and opinions were often apparently curiously coloured by their owner's isolation. It was as though his disorder had forced him to become a bystander in the business of living, starving him of social relationships and of the most basic human experiences. All things intrigued him: descriptions of meetings, places, people, occasions; there was nothing that failed to arouse in him a wistful curiosity.

As the curtains screening Joseph's personality were slowly drawn aside, Treves discovered how many of his impressions of the world came not from first-hand knowledge but rather from books. He was an avid reader, having learnt to read as a child, and books had been a constant source of solace in his loneliness. His knowledge of literature was both eccentric and diverse, for his selection of reading matter had been determined more by what chance brought to hand than by consciously exploring or developing reading tastes. He had simply devoured anything that presented itself: the Bible and the Prayer Book several times, so that he knew both intimately. He had an extensive acquaintance with newspapers and magazines of all kinds, even a patchy knowledge of the works of more serious novelists, including Jane Austen. He had struggled with a string of lesson books and enjoyed a host of stories. In fact he had read and considered any scrap of writing that fell into his hands.

Whenever he discussed his reading, the void his books had filled and the reality they took on in his mind soon became apparent. He was apt to speak of novels as if they were factual accounts not fictional narratives. He described plots as though they were events that had happened recently, recounted conversations in animated detail and spoke of characters as if they possessed lives of their own, discussing their plights and predicaments with sincere concern. Through taking his books into his head, he thus led a kind of surrogate life to parallel his own realities and compensate to some extent for the denial to him of experiences in the real world.

At such moments, watching his excitement and involvement, Frederick Treves realized that Merrick possessed unguessed-at emotional depths; that beneath the grave and rather hesitant courtesy lay a turmoil of emotions. Joseph could be moved to excitement and agitation, even compassion and grief, as easily as a child, but in his case the stirring up of feelings was powerful, profound and lasting. The discovery of such fundamental and easily provoked emotions in his patient was something that both startled and disturbed Treves.

From his reading Joseph therefore derived most of his impressions of human nature, having had few opportunities to study people closely. He had met men from many walks of life and in wide varieties of circumstance: idle sightseers, doctors, music-hall entrepreneurs, Poor Law officials, showmen, policemen, workhouse keepers, surgeons. From them he had received wide varieties of treatment and reaction, unkind, kind and professional. His ideal of manhood meanwhile remained a strangely compounded creature. It was derived in part from novels with descriptions of the manly virtues of heroes drawn, it seemed, almost exclusively from the aristocracy and living lives of idle luxury; in part from the advertisement columns of the newspapers, with their emphases on such necessary accessories to the outward show of a gentleman as travelling bags, patent-leather shoes or dressing cases. It was a vision of the romantic hero, though as the rather demanding ideal of a gentleman it bore little resemblance to men he had actually met.

His image of the opposite sex was even more difficult, and several degrees more intense. But his attitude to women might be defined in the most simple terms: he felt an admiration bordering on idolatry. Perhaps with somewhat ominous undertones, he confided to Treves that his favourite reading consisted of stories dealing with love and romance.

At the age of seventeen, Joseph had been admitted to the segregated wards of the workhouse; at twenty-one, he emerged into the carefully screened-off world of the showman's booth; for the past seven years, the pattern of his life had been practically monastic. Women were an enigma, a totally unknown quantity, and his vision of womanhood was largely an amalgamation made up from his books, his imagination and the transcending memory of his mother.

Women were thus creatures to be set apart, beings of a gentler and purer spirit. He saw each one as the heroine of some untold story, a person to be regarded with such reverence and awe that she must be unapproachable, let alone obtainable. Women were and should be as they existed in the pages of romantic chivalry: delicate, more finely moulded creatures than men, needing to be protected, cherished but above all worshipped.

It was the image to which he clung throughout his life, even though it was cruelly at odds with his experience. His actual encounters with women had been associated with pain and distress. Invariably in any woman whom he met there would be immediate and obvious signs of shock and revulsion. In some cases the reaction was so extreme that they screamed and ran away, even fainted on the spot. Only from the matron of the London Hospital,

Miss Eva Lückes, and her nursing staff did he receive unflinching courtesy and consideration, but even here there was a sense of a certain instinctive constraint. They were, he recognized, but nurses carrying out a necessary duty in a professional way.

While Joseph now had rooms of his own, the burden of nursing him remained no light matter; and in spite of the care lavished on him, his day-to-day life was far from easy. His condition continued to grow more troublesome; his hip was painful, his movements slow and stubborn. The weight of his enlarged limbs tired him quickly and he found it impossible to perform many small tasks on his own account. Even in bed it was difficult for him to rest since he found it impossible to lie flat. Should he do so, the weight of the fleshy and bony growths on his skull made it unmanageable and he was overcome by a sensation of the head rolling backwards, stretching and constricting the neck muscles. To sleep, he found it essential to continue to crouch upright on the bed in a foetal parody, his legs drawn up, his arms clasped about them and his heavy head resting on his knees.

There were occasions when Treves found himself peering in on something of the boredom and loneliness to which Joseph was essentially condemned all his life. At certain periods Joseph became hopelessly despondent. For hours at a time, when he thought himself unobserved, he might sit staring before him, beating slowly and rhythmically on his pillow or the arm of his chair with his deformed right arm. It seemed to Treves that Joseph was keeping time to a tune heard only in his mind – one which he was unable to voice, for he could never attempt to whistle or even sing. The surgeon saw the habit as an expression of inward cheerfulness, but a trained observer today would rather interpret it as a classic depressive symptom.

Once, during such a period of depression, Joseph startled Treves by returning to the subject of his future care. It was clear that he had still not grasped that the new quarters were his to occupy for life. Some of the suggestions members of the public had made when Carr Gomm launched the appeal found an echo in his own thoughts, for he inquired about the time when he would have to move on, suggesting that he might perhaps find a refuge in some out-of-the-way spot, such as a lighthouse or an asylum for the blind. It was a distressing task trying to convince this small and infinitely vulnerable man that he had no need to journey further.

But Treves was also coming to realize that Joseph's sanctuary in the basement rooms was in danger of turning into a prison. Joseph's sense of isolation was increasing and Treves felt certain that much of his patient's distress sprang from the loneliness life had forced on him. To Treves it seemed that these sufferings came at least in part from having been rejected by so many fellow human beings. More than anything else, he felt it necessary to convince Joseph that he could be accepted on equal terms as a normal person. One possible solution might be to introduce him to people who would disregard his hideous appearance and communicate with him with courtesy and consideration. For this particular task, who more suitable than a well-bred lady of the British upper middle class, versed in composure and social virtue? Yet the failure of such an experiment might well turn into irreparable disaster. Treves cast about in his mind for such a person who might be persuaded to meet Merrick and who could be relied upon to be strong-minded enough to keep her nerve whatever her inner feelings.

At last, Treves said, he asked a friend, 'a young and pretty widow, if she thought she could enter Merrick's room with a smile, wish him good morning and shake him by the hand'. It was essential that she should betray no trace of revulsion or embarrassment. The young widow whom Treves approached was Mrs Leila Maturin, who had lost her husband, Dr Leslie Maturin, in 1883 within only two months of their marriage. She listened to Treves's proposal and his description of the Elephant Man. Then, without hesitation, she accepted the role in which he cast her: an introduction of beauty to the beast, though with strict limits on the hopes of a transformation.

Treves accompanied Leila Maturin as she was taken to the little basement room to meet Joseph. She entered with an easy grace, smiling as she approached, reaching out and taking his hand as Treves presented him.

It was all too much. Speech was beyond him. Slowly he released her hand and slowly he bent his great head forward to his knees as he broke into heart-rending sobs and wept uncontrollably. The meeting ended as quickly as it had begun.

Afterwards Joseph confided to a rather shaken Treves that it was the first time any strange woman had smiled at him, let alone taken his hand in greeting. The event itself turned out to be a landmark, ushering in a wholly new phase in the life of the Elephant Man. Treves pinpointed it as the moment when a renewal of self-confidence began for Joseph Merrick. The old hurts and haunting fears of spying eyes and whispered wonderings slowly began to heal and dissolve. The impulse to hide himself from the world was transformed into a renewed curiosity and a wish to reach out to grasp some of the small everyday experiences that were commonplace in the lives of ordinary people but hitherto as beyond Joseph's reach as if they had something to do with life on the moon.

After this time Treves gained the impression that Joseph fell in love with every attractive woman he met – though 'in a humble and devotional way', he was careful to qualify. Treves's thoroughness in ensuring that no mirror came his way in which he might catch a chance glimpse of himself meanwhile led Joseph to forget the full horror of his appearance. 'He was amorous,' said Treves. 'He would like to have been a lover, to have walked with the beloved object in the languorous shades of some beautiful garden and to have poured into her ear all the glowing utterances that he had rehearsed in his heart.' Treves sensed that behind Merrick's speculative musings over finding a refuge in an asylum for the blind was the idea that he might raise a spark of affection in the heart of some blind girl who could not see the disfigurement of his flesh.

Such thoughts were clearly safer left sublimated in the realms of romantic chivalry. Treves was a directly robust character among Victorian doctors, a scientific realist as well as a man of imagination. The sharp irony of the fact that Joseph's genitalia remained perfectly normal among all his deformities cannot have been beyond him.

CHAPTER 9

'Such a Gentle, Kindly Man, Poor Thing!'

Even during the early days following his admission to the London Hospital, the case of Joseph Merrick began to attract the attention of people who were in a position to bring social influence to bear on his behalf. Outstanding among these was the actress, Mrs Kendal, to whose actor husband, W. H. Kendal, Mr Wardell Cardew mentioned the fact of Joseph Merrick having been in Ostend. Wardell Cardew went on to suggest that Mr Kendal might care to go to the London Hospital to see the Elephant Man for himself, and so he did. In fact Kendal had studied medicine for a time before deciding to make his career in the theatre, and among his friends was John Bland-Sutton. He had made a point of keeping up his interest in medical topics.

When he returned home his wife asked him whether he had enjoyed himself amid all the medical activity. According to her memoirs, *Dame Madge Kendal by Herself*, he replied decisively:

'No . . . I have not. I have seen the most fearful sight of my life.'

'Don't tell me about it,' I replied.

'The extraordinary thing,' declared my husband, 'is that out of the distorted frame came the most musical voice.'

The experience so affected him that he could hardly speak. When he recovered, he told me that Mr Cardew had said they would never allow Merrick to be in the hospital permanently, although he ought to be in there, as it was not fit that he should be seen in public.

'Wouldn't they let him remain in the hospital,' I asked, 'if the money was raised to pay for his keep?'

At this time Madge Kendal was appearing at the St James's Theatre, Piccadilly, with her husband's business partner in theatrical management, Mr John Hare, in *The Hobby Horse*, a new play by the rising young playwright Arthur Pinero. The fine cast also included Mrs Beerbohm Tree, and the drama critic of *Punch* said he really did not care in what Mrs Kendal and Mr Hare appeared, they excelled so in their playing. Evidently the play was not vintage Pinero, but Mrs Kendal had the rewarding and appropriate part of an irreproachable married woman whose one peculiarity was her philanthropic hobby of turning the family house into a refuge for waifs and strays, to her husband's exasperation. It was a success with the theatre-going public, for whom Mrs Kendal was a star performer and could do no wrong.

Madge Kendal had been born into a family with strong theatrical antecedents, the Robertsons. Among her ancestors was James Robertson, an actor and playwright who was a contemporary of David Garrick and well known in the fashionable centres of Bath and York. Several generations of theatrical managers followed, and one of her elder brothers (there were twenty-two children in the family) was T. W. Robertson, the dramatist who had a decisive influence in introducing the new realism on to the Victorian stage. He saw this as a principle that would affect a production as a whole, from playscript to style of the acting and production details. He was one of the first to stipulate that when he asked for coat-pegs in the scenery they should be real coat-pegs on which real coats might be hung and not painted simulations.

When Madge Robertson married W. H. Kendal in 1869, her career as an accomplished and popular actress was already firmly launched. Her husband was similarly becoming well known as an actor manager, though in the end it was his wife's fame that was the more durable. Nevertheless their partnership lasted throughout their lives and they became a byword for setting a respectable example in the theatrical world where a general raffishness characterized the more usual tone.

All her life Madge Kendal never flinched from performing acts of charity. Many years after the events concerning the Elephant Man she was to claim that she had been the one responsible for anonymously launching the fund that brought Merrick the financial security to maintain him in the London Hospital. Be that as it may, it needs to be emphasized that while her husband met Merrick, she herself probably never did so. The chapter on 'The Elephant Man' in her memoirs contains no indication of a personal encounter. The tone is detached and she even relies on Treves's already published description to sketch in his appearance. Her incessantly crowded career could, in any case, have left her little enough time for charitable visits in the manner of ladies of greater leisure.

She nevertheless represented the starting point to a network of personages who would mobilize sympathy for Joseph Merrick's welfare and incidentally enrich his experience of a social life in the few years remaining to him. In the meantime, he had begun to explore within the limits he could manage: a few limping steps in the darkness of late evening, a shuffling from his room, a painful toiling up the concrete steps and then the cold stillness of Bedstead Square with its shadows, the far-away glow of the high ward windows and the occasional echo of distant footsteps. Yet it prompted in him a sense of freedom to stand unmolested in the open air. With each night-time excursion, his confidence increased until at last he was able to make his way from the square, skirting beyond the patches of light thrown from windows, picking his way through the rubble of builders' materials that littered the ground where new extensions were being built, moving in a hesitant exploration round beyond the end of the great block of the East Wing until he came to the hospital gardens and walked alone in the darkness. There he could feel the grass soft beneath his feet and savour the rediscovered scent of night flowers.

In the daytime, he spied cautiously on the comings and goings in Bedstead Square. He learnt to recognize the faces of those who passed daily above his window, and the workmen in their turn were aware of the unseen but watchful presence behind the curtains in the little basement room. Here, too, he unexpectedly found friends. Mr Taylor, the chief engineer, came one day to introduce Charles Taylor, his youngest son, a lad of about seventeen. A friendship quickly sprang up between them, and after that the youth came regularly, bringing his violin to play in private recital for Joseph's entertainment.

Mrs Kendal sent him gifts, the first being an early gramophone of the type invented by Edison only about ten years before, the recordings for which were made on cylinders rotated by a hand-cranked handle at the side. Joseph wrote to thank Mrs Kendal for her kindness, and in fact he wrote her letters on several occasions. Alas, the letters did not survive. She presented them to the London Hospital, but they could no longer be traced when she came to write her memoirs in the early 1930s. He also sent her one of the cardboard models he had constructed with the aid of the nurses. It was a delicately detailed model of a Gothic church. This has survived, being preserved today in the museum of the London Hospital Medical College.

In one of his letters to Mrs Kendal, Joseph mentioned that he hoped one day to be able to learn basket-work. She promptly arranged for an instructor to teach him the craft. Now his room became littered with bundles of cane and small basket-work articles waiting to be given to whoever might accept them. The first basket he completed he sent to Mrs Kendal herself.

Since it was evidently not possible for her to go to see him, Joseph requested that she send him some photographs. These she forwarded, and he displayed them in his room in triumph.

It came as rather a surprise to Treves to find how Joseph was starting to develop into something of a celebrity. The letter to *The Times* had had the effect of arousing not only a phenomenal charitable response but also widespread curiosity. Requests to visit the Elephant Man were received by the hospital. Within a few months of the disturbing incident of his meeting with the pretty young widow, Treves came to the rueful conclusion that every lady of note in the social sphere would soon make the pilgrimage to the hospital to be escorted to the basement rooms and introduced. Each one who came was forewarned about his appearance, and each one sturdily summoned the courage to greet him with smile and handshake, even to spend some minutes in conversation.

To begin with, Joseph was reticent towards his guests, but every introduction seemed to bring him a little more confidence, and each day his manner became more self-assured. Treves still needed to act as interpreter. Joseph's speech was improving with practice but it remained indistinct. His visitors, though perhaps drawn mainly by curiosity or the fact that it was fast becoming the done thing to visit Joseph Merrick, were entirely benevolent. They brought him gifts so that his rooms grew bright with ornaments and pictures. Sometimes he received autographed portraits or photographs of the ladies who called, and these joined the others displayed about the room. Some of the gentlemen left money to be spent on his behalf, and in this Treves acted as steward. The gifts that always pleased Joseph most were books, for he was slowly accumulating quite a respectable library and his spare time was increasingly given to reading.

The paradox was not lost on Treves as he saw Joseph emerging into an object of patronage and interest. His protégé, once a homeless and shunned waif, was beginning to become the sought after acquaintance of duchesses and countesses. It is doubtful, however, whether the surgeon could have taken the irony the one step further, and have seen the accident of his own intervention as carrying Joseph's career as a freak on to a new, unimaginable level of success; or himself as the *alter ego* to Mr Tom Norman, the showman he so consistently despised.

As Joseph lost the last of his reticence, he would speak relaxedly and strike up acquaintanceship with anyone who paused to acknowledge him. It became his habit to sit at his window to have a word with whoever happened to pass in Bedstead Square. He no longer hung back behind the curtains, and regular passers-by often stopped and called to inspect his more recent gifts or hear tales of the distinguished guests he had entertained. Such tales were told with an innocent jubilation, steeped more in wonder than in pride. On a few occasions he wandered away from his room in search of company, and once raised an alarm by appearing without warning at the entrance to one of the main wards. Only a flurry of nurses rushing to gather about him and shepherd him back to his own quarters prevented his sudden presence delivering a shock to the other patients.

Joseph's fresh curiosity about the outside world naturally extended to Treves. He questioned the surgeon shyly about himself and the home where he and his family lived. He seemed particularly inquisitive about the house, asking wistfully about its arrangement and how it looked. At last he remarked obliquely that he should like to see the inside of a 'real' house. The simple artisan terrace dwellings, such as he knew in Leicester, or the lodgings of the freakshow circuit, could never have counted as such. It was the elegant town houses of the rich, as he had glimpsed them standing splendid and remote during his travels, their doors perpetually closed, which teased his imagination. With the help of his reading he had been able to people and furnish their splendid interiors, but now he wanted to measure imagined images against the facts.

Treves recognized the wish implied by Joseph's mention of the subject. Within a few days he arranged for him to be taken to his own house at 6 Wimpole Street, safely concealed inside a hansom cab. No doubt the household was suitably prepared, and Treves's daughters, Enid, aged eight, and Hetty, aged four, safely out of the way when Joseph was hurried across the pavements and into the seclusion of the hallway.

Solemnly Treves escorted his guest from room to room. It turned out to be a slow process, for Joseph paused to examine every object. He gazed at each piece of furniture, each curtain, each fabric with almost comically exaggerated interest. As they progressed, Treves became aware of a sense of unease within himself. The house seemed in some way to be falling short of expectations. Joseph had clearly anticipated finding a larger and grander establishment and was puzzled by the lack of liveried footmen and other servants in attendance. (Treves himself, when writing of his consulting room, once described it as the smallest in London, 'not much more than a cupboard with a fireplace and window'.)

Anxious that Joseph should not be disappointed, while hoping to explain circumstances and perhaps retrieve a certain lost prestige, Treves explained that this was never meant to be the home of an aristocrat. It was more accurately a town house, built in the more modest style of dwellings as described in the novels of Jane Austen. Joseph, who had read *Emma*, accepted the comparison with polite gravity.

From the time of its foundation in the eighteenth century, the London Hospital was forced to wage a continuous battle against not only lack of funds but also a shortage of accommodation. In 1887 two sets of new buildings were nearing completion. On the south side of Bedstead Square, beyond the end of the East Wing, the new Nurses Home was being constructed. In Turner Street, at the side of the hospital, new accommodation for the Medical College was almost finished. By the spring of 1887, both buildings were completed, and on 21 May the official opening was held.

The Prince and Princess of Wales accepted the invitation to perform the ceremony, and their carriage arrived at the main gates at five in the afternoon on a day wet with a steady drizzle. They were received by a formal reception party headed by the president of the London Hospital, George William, second Duke of Cambridge, Commander in Chief of the Army and a cousin of Queen Victoria's.

As a young man of twenty-one, George William had defied the conventions expected of a royal duke by marrying a commoner who was worse still an actress. His successful life-long marriage was quietly ignored by the monarch, the court and society at large. He had been on active service during the Crimean War, and had his horse shot from under him at the battle of Inkerman, though he then managed to rally a hundred survivors from the division to break through the encircling Russians. By the 1880s the veteran warrior was ageing and gruffly formidable. He had as good as inherited the presidency of the hospital from his father, who died in 1850, and was untiring in the support he offered and rallied. He graced official occasions, spoke at innumerable dinners, presided over charitable gatherings and maintained a determined supervision of the hospital's variegated activities. He never hesitated to voice displeasure should someone omit to consult him over some important piece of institutional business, though his irascibility was in general recognized as concealing genuine concern and kindness. He had even continued to meet these commitments during the years of Queen Victoria's retirement from public life after the death of the Prince Consort in 1861, when he shouldered many of the public tasks expected from the head of state.

The Prince and Princess of Wales had themselves kept up an association with the London Hospital since 1864. One of their joint duties in that year, which followed the year of their marriage, had been to lay the foundation stone for the new block known as the Alexandra Wing. For 21 May 1887, the plans were more elaborate. The royal party would first be conducted to the new Nurses Home, to be received in the dining-room by the matron, Miss Eva Lückes, heading her nursing staff. The chapel choir would then sing a hymn, the suffragan Bishop of Bedford would read a collect and the Duke of Cambridge would ask the Princess of Wales to declare the building, to be called the Alexandra Home, open. From there the party would be escorted to the new Medical College buildings, where further speeches would be delivered and a similar ceremony performed by the Prince of Wales; but on the way the royal personages would be invited to visit several wards.

The slow, dignified procession duly passed from bed to bed, and the princess was visibly moved by the spectacle of so much suffering. Then, from the wards, the party descended to the basements of the East Wing so that she might be introduced to the Elephant Man, who had by that time been almost a year in residence. She was warned that his appearance was literally shocking, and Frederick Treves accompanied the party as a matter of course.

Thus Joseph Merrick suddenly found his small room flooded with strangers, but for him the most important person among them was the Princess of Wales. She had entered the room with relaxed grace, smiled and taken the introduction with perfect serenity, shaken him by the hand and sat beside his chair so she might talk to him. She examined his curios and gifts with an interest that left him transported with wonder. The Prince of Wales also spoke to him, being quietly amused to spot Mrs Kendal among the collection of autographed portraits. And then the royal party withdrew, leaving Joseph beside himself with excitement.

Later that night, the Duke of Cambridge confided to his diary some details of the afternoon:

> 1887, May 21st – Went to the London Hospital, where as President I received at 5 o'clock the Prince and Princess of Wales, who came to open the new home just finished for the Nurses of the Hospital. We passed through the wards, saw the unfortunate man called the elephant man, who is a painful sight to look at, though intelligent in himself, and then I read an address to the Prince and Princess to which the Prince replied. It was very wet, but we were able to return in

open carriages. The crowds in the streets were very enthusiastic. All went off well.

It was probably on this occasion, though he did not mention it, that the Duke of Cambridge discreetly presented Joseph with a silver watch.

The following afternoon he paid a call on his mother, the aged Duchess of Cambridge. Lady Geraldine Somerset, who attended the duchess, kept a journal for her, and in this she recorded the duke's visit:

May 22nd, 1887
... At 3 came the Duke. He gave H.R.H. an account ... of the Princess of Wales ... at the London Hospital, tearing up her bouquet, to give a flower of it to each sick child & each sick woman. Of their having seen the Elephant-man, poor creature – a sad spectacle! *enormous*, with two great bosses on the forehead really like an elephant's head, & a protruding face like a snout, one *enormous* hand like the foot of an elephant, the other, the left hand, extraordinarily, exceptionally *small*! He can never go out, he is mobbed so, & lives therefore a prisoner; he is less disgusting to see than might be, because he is such a gentle, kindly man, poor thing! ...

The Duke of Cambridge clearly put across a graphic account of Joseph to his mother. On his side Joseph treasured the memory of the meeting, recounting the events over and over, though the excitement was not yet done with. Before long he received a small package from Marlborough House. It contained a signed photograph of the Princess of Wales, sent so he might include it in his collection. For Joseph, whose emotions lay constantly just below the surface, the gift was overwhelming, and he broke down and wept over it. It was so important to him that he could scarcely bear even Treves to touch it. It was framed for him, and he hung it in his room, treating it almost as an icon.

Treves suggested he should write to the princess to thank her, and he did so, naïvely beginning his letter, 'My dear Princess' and signing it off, 'Yours very sincerely'. When asked by Joseph to read the letter to see if it was all right, Treves was so touched that he let it go as it stood. The princess visited Joseph on other occasions, and when Christmas came sent him not one but three Christmas cards, each one personally inscribed with a message on the back. A further effect of her interest was to amplify the volume of other illustrious visitors. 'It became a cult among the personal friends of the Princess,' wrote John Bland-Sutton, 'to visit the Elephant Man in the London Hospital.' Neither did the Prince of Wales forget him. From time to time a bag of game would arrive for Joseph's table following a shoot on the royal estates.

Some years later, at a charity garden fête given by Sir William Treloar in Chelsea, Mrs Kendal was selling autographed photographs of herself at one of the stalls. The former Prince of Wales, by now King Edward VII, surveyed each picture in turn before solemnly informing her, 'I think, Mrs Kendal, you must have given your best photographs to James Merrick.' Evidently something King Edward and Frederick Treves had in common was a difficulty with the Elephant Man's correct Christian name.

Christmas at the London Hospital was always a well-observed festival. For weeks beforehand the nursing staff prepared decorations for the wards; for days gifts poured in at the main gates. Festivities began quietly in the early hours of Christmas morning when a choir of sisters and nurses moved from ward to ward, singing carols. Then, during the morning, Father Christmas himself arrived, helped by an assorted band of fairies to distribute a present to every patient.

At midday, as the resident doctors carved the turkeys in the lobbies to each of their wards, the patients settled down to a special dinner sanctioned by the house committee. This was finished off with a slice of plum pudding. For the sisters, nurses and probationers there were special dinners enriched with delicacies provided by the senior surgeons and physicians. In the afternoon, the consultant staff came with their children to watch the shows, for the residents, nurses, students and dentals then dressed up to tour the hospital and perform amateur entertainments for the patients. For the children there was a Punch and Judy show. In the evening, as the wards settled into darkness, a Christmas dance was given for the wardmaids, and later there was a midnight supper for the scrubbers.

The coming of Christmas for Joseph Merrick meant, in the first place, the arrival of his Christmas cards – not only the polite cards from nurses and staff but those from the various visitors who had befriended him, including the ones from Princess Alexandra. There were also many personal gifts.

One year, shortly before Christmas, Treves asked Joseph what he felt he would like, for several donations of money had been handed in for his benefit. Joseph showed no hesitation. He had seen an advertisement for a gentleman's dressing case with silver fittings that appealed to him so much he had kept the cutting from the newspaper. The set consisted of silver-backed hairbrushes and comb, a silver shoehorn and a hat brush as well as ivory-handled razors and toothbrushes. It seemed an incongruous choice, but Treves understood the feelings behind it and purchased the set at once. He intervened only to prepare the gift by removing the mirror and carefully filling the cigarette case with cigarettes, though he knew Joseph never smoked and never could with his deformed lips; but then every item in the case was equally useless to him in any utilitarian sense.

The dressing case turned out to be the perfect prop for Joseph's imagination. In the privacy of his small room, sitting quietly as he arranged its contents, opening and closing the cigarette case, he became an elegant, sophisticated man-about-town, preparing in his dressing-room for some formal dinner or glittering occasion.

By now Treves was beginning positively to relish introducing Joseph to new experiences. There was, he found, something about it of the pleasure to be derived from watching a child's astonishment when surprised by a fresh and unexpected wonder. Among Joseph's unfulfilled social aspirations was to enjoy an evening out at a West End theatre, but the difficulties here were immense. Any audience that caught a glimpse of Joseph Merrick among them was hardly to be expected to pay much further attention to anything on the stage. The matter reached the ears of Mrs Kendal, who saw at once that the answer could be for Joseph to watch the stage from a position of concealment. She moved to exploit her social contacts and went to call on the Baroness Burdett-Coutts.

The baroness, who kept a private box in the Theatre Royal, Drury Lane, was among the richest women in nineteenth-century England. She was a notable philanthropist, a patroness of the arts and of the theatre in particular, who had set up Henry Irving for his famous period of occupancy at the Lyceum Theatre. Now in her seventies, she still held a controlling interest in Coutts, the bankers founded by her grandfather, and so was banker to the royal family. Both the first Duke and Duchess of Cambridge were her friends, as was the second duke, the president of the London Hospital. Guests as diverse as the Duke of Wellington, Sir Robert Peel, Samuel Wilberforce, W. E. Gladstone and Benjamin Disraeli had dined at her table.

She was formidably well informed, cultivating, as well as politicians, scientists such as Michael Faraday and Joseph Hooker, or writers such as Charles Dickens, who gave her the dedication to *Martin Chuzzlewit*. She helped to finance the expeditions to Africa of David Livingstone, and later those of Henry Morton Stanley. Her vast fortune was used for prodigious acts of charity in which, while he was alive, Dickens would advise her.

The baroness had made her private box at Drury Lane available to many people in the past, including Dickens and his family, but the prospect of the Elephant Man occupying it caused her misgivings. What, she asked, would the dreadful effect be if an unfortunate woman unexpectedly caught sight of him? The consequences could be unimaginable. Mrs Kendal assured the baroness that arrangements would lie in the capable hands of Frederick Treves, that no one would see the Elephant Man arrive at or leave the theatre, and that care would be taken to ensure he was in no way visible to the audience. The baroness withdrew her objections and plans for the operation were set in motion.

It was by now the pantomime season at Drury Lane, the Christmas pantomime being a firmly established tradition in the Victorian theatre. The famous sequence of annual pantomimes at Drury Lane that Augustus Harris mounted there after he took over its management in 1880 had become bywords for rich and elaborate spectacle as well as the use of star names from the London music halls to play the leads. As *The Times* critic remarked in 1883:

On the stage commanded by Augustus Harris the tales of Fairyland are annually illustrated with a magnificence which sets criticism at nought. They hardly fall within the domain of drama. They are a dream, a phantasmagoria, the baseless fabric of a vision, and are best appreciated in a spirit of child-like wonderment.

Neither Treves nor Madge Kendal tell us which of those famous productions it was planned for Joseph to see, but the year Joseph Merrick was taken to Drury Lane with Madge Kendal's help can only have been 1887. It could not have been the previous year, since the business of Joseph's admission to the London Hospital was then only just being resolved. From the summer of 1888, the movements and preoccupations of the Kendals make it unlikely that Mrs Kendal could have been available in London to assist. On 21 July 1888, the long partnership between the Kendals and Mr John Hare at the St James's Theatre finally broke up. With *The Weaker Sex*, a new play by Arthur Pinero, under their wings, the Kendals established a company of their own. There were problems to be ironed out in the play's presentation and, to run it in, they took it on a tour of the provinces.

Their first night was at Manchester on 28 September 1888. Not till six months later did they bring the production to London, opening at the Court Theatre on 16 March 1889. They stayed at the Court Theatre throughout the summer, planning their first great tour of the United States. By the autumn they had left England, opening triumphantly at the Fifth Avenue Theatre, New York, in October 1889. They did not then return to England until 26 June 1890.

Had Joseph seen the show of 1888 he would have witnessed the début in pantomime of the great comedian Dan Leno in *The Babes in the Wood*. But the production he saw was *Puss in Boots*, a deduction confirmed by the fact that the pamphlet *The Elephant Man* was published in 1888 (see Appendix Two, page 176). It is doubtful anyway whether he would have been appreciative of Dan Leno, the element of the comedians holding little appeal for him.

The book for *Puss in Boots* was written by E. L. Blanchard, who scripted every pantomime at Drury Lane between 1852 and 1888 and had in his day been responsible for giving the *genre* a certain literary quality. Each year under Augustus Harris's management, however, Blanchard complained ever more bitterly at the way his scripts were ruthlessly reworked to make room for some ambitious scenic procession or the comic business of the music-hall artists. The tradition was changing and Blanchard was powerless to do anything except grouse, as he once did in his diary: '. . . hardly anything done as I intended it, or spoken as I had written: the music-hall element is crushing out the rest and the good old fairy-tales never again to be illustrated as they should be.' In fact Harris was giving the public of the 1880s what it wanted, and his panto-mimes usually justified the lavish financial investments that went into mounting them.

Such considerations would not have had even an academic interest for Joseph. The whole affair was to turn out to be for him an experience of unexampled wonder from the moment he was smuggled into Drury Lane Theatre from a carriage with drawn blinds. Permission was given to use the royal entrance with its private staircase, and, 'All went well,' said Treves, 'and no one saw a figure, more monstrous than any on the stage, mount the staircase or cross the corridor.' Once in the private box, a trio of ward sisters wearing normal evening dress who had volunteered for the job, sat in the front row to create a human screen. Treves then sat with Joseph effectively concealed in the shadows at the back.

To realize Joseph's feelings at that moment would need a total recall of the biggest treat of childhood, before the encroachment of experience made such absorptions of innocent uncritical vision impossible. Under the direction of Mr Jimmy Glover, the resident conductor, the theatre band struck up the overture, and the curtain rose on the opening scene. Mr Blanchard kept his story line close to the fairy-tale Charles Perrault had made familiar to generations of children. It was one of those included in the collection of nursery tales he made in the seventeenth century, the *Contes de ma mère l'Oye*, though it had far more ancient origins in Italian folk story.

The youngest son of a miller inherits, when his father dies, nothing but the cat. In company with his feline friend, he sets out to seek his fortune in the world. One day, while he is swimming, a royal coach approaches and the quick-witted cat cries out to it to stop, for, it says, his master is drowning. Dragged from the water the bewildered youth finds himself introduced by the cat to the King, Queen and Princess as the Marquis of Carabas. Afterwards the boy and his cat travel to an ogre's castle, where the cat tricks the monster into turning himself first into a lion, then into a mouse; whereupon he falls on him and eats him up. Having thus taken possession of the ogre's castle, lands and treasure, the cat presents them to his master to make him a fit match for the princess of the realm. The young couple, needless to say, had already fallen in love when their eyes first engaged.

For Augustus Harris the simple scaffolding of the traditional tale provided a springboard for a variety of extravagances, not all of which had much to do with advancing the story. The list of performers was long. There were the music-hall songs, the balletic interludes, the harlequinade and the climax of the transformation scene all to be incorporated. The part of Jocelyn, the miller's son, otherwise known as the Marquis of Carabas, was taken by Miss Tilly Wadman as principal boy, 'handsome and plays and sings charmingly', according to *Punch*, though *The Times* felt her singing 'was not always very true, but she makes a capital Burlesque Prince'. Master Charles Lauri took the part of Puss, while another popular animal parody act was the tightrope-walking Blondin Donkey of the Brothers Griffiths. Letty Lind, a rising star among the dancing girls of the Gaiety Theatre who had made her début there only that year, was the Princess Sweetheart.

'Neatly tripping, lightly dancing Letty Lind,' enthused *The Times*, 'who has already made herself a favourite with the children and their attendants.' 'These are leggy days,' said *Punch* more cryptically.

The part of the King was taken by Herbert Campbell, a comic singer from the music halls who came to specialize in dame parts, though not on this occasion. The Queen was played by Harry Nicholls, a light comedy actor.

> The one [said *The Times*] is a pantomime monarch worthy of Thackeray in *The Rose and the Ring*, and the other a depressed but loquacious Queen who manages to get in more than one

word edgeways. All the matrimonial squabbles, all the domestic wrangling, all the polite sarcasms and family jars are conceived in the best spirit of humour by two actors who are singularly observant ... The fun they get out of the journey in the stage coach, the incident of the pretended drowning of the Marquis of Carabas, and the struggle for supremacy with the costermonger's donkey [the well-known 'Blondin Donkey' animal impersonation of the Brothers Griffiths], are all in the best and most legitimate spirit of pantomime fun.

The harlequinade towards the end was, of course, a link back to the very origins of pantomime burlesque, and by now almost anachronistic in the changing tradition. The leading part of the clown was in this case taken by Mr Harry Payne, resident clown in the Drury Lane pantomimes from 1883 until 1894, the year before his death. Prior to this he used to play Harlequin, and his father, W. H. Payne, had worked as a pantomimist with the great Grimaldi.

But, said Treves, Merrick 'did not like the ogres and the giants, while the funny men impressed him as irreverent. Having no experience as a boy of romping and ragging, or practical jokes and "larks", he had little sympathy with the doings of the clown ...' On the other hand he reacted with pleasure when the policeman's dignity was decisively undermined by being smacked about the face and knocked backwards. Whatever he may have witnessed of police officiousness towards the freakshows was no doubt a factor in his response. For the rest it was the spectacle that entranced him.

His reaction was not so much that of delight as of wonder and amazement. He was awed. He was enthralled. The spectacle left him speechless, so that if he were spoken to he took no heed. He often seemed to be panting for breath ... [he was] thrilled by a vision that was almost beyond his comprehension ... The splendour and display impressed him, but, I think, the ladies of the ballet took a still greater hold on his fancy.

Three 'Spectacular Scenes' punctuated Augustus Harris's ambitious production, two of them, according to *The Times*, being 'veritable dreams of beauty'. The first showed the inner court of the King and Queen's palace: '. . . a dazzling structure of marble, with high raised galleries, lofty columns and a grand staircase down which a dozen people can walk abreast'. And down the staircase tripped chambermaids in yellow and blue gowns, followed by a procession, heralded by trumpeters, of the entire court in costumes that exhausted 'the whole catalogue of colours'. The *Illustrated London News* was carried into transports of exclaiming that bits of the production were 'worthy of Paolo Veronese'.

The second great spectacle came after the pantomime cat had cunningly disposed of the ogre. The vast hall of the ogre's castle was suddenly seen to be 'filled with warriors in complete armour', some mounted, others on foot. These forces launched themselves into an elaborate drill routine with halberds, whereupon a great expanse of tapestry at the back was drawn aside to reveal yet another staircase, down which swarmed

> . . . some countless warriors in gold and silver armour fol-
> lowed by knights accompanied by their squires and standard
> bearers. The entire stage in its length and breadth is filled
> with glittering metal, nodding plumes and fluttering pennons
> which rival in colour the whole tribe of butterflies.

The third and last spectacle was that against which the fairy ballet took place and that became the transformation scene. In the foreground was an oak glade, the boughs of whose mighty trees overarched the stage, their trunks surrounded by a rich array of fern and foxglove. Beyond the glade stretched a lake, golden in summer light and surrounded by more trees. A line of distant hills on the backcloth closed the enchanted vista. The object of it all, said the *Illustrated London News*, was

> . . . to present, by means of children and girls, a wedding
> bouquet. It is charmingly and fancifully carried out, and the
> most delightful result of white flowers and green leaves,
> maidenhair fern, roses, lilies, stephanotis, daisies and azalea
> is attained at minimum cost.

For some reason the culminating scene, meant to out-dazzle all that had gone before, was felt to fall rather flat. But it was placed at the end of an evening that had already stretched far into the night. Indeed, the fatigued critic of *Punch* suggested the pantomime might, next year, be drastically curtailed so the audience could rely on leaving for home by 11 p.m. Yet the opinions of critics played no part in Joseph Merrick's responses. So far as he was concerned it could have gone on for ever. For Frederick Treves, on the other hand, it must have marked the end of a very long day indeed, since he had no doubt risen as usual at five in the morning. He still, moreover, had the responsibility of smuggling Joseph back out of the theatre and into his closed carriage before escorting him safely home to Whitechapel.

Time did nothing to fade the glow of Joseph Merrick's bewitchment during the weeks that followed. He would talk of the pantomime continually, and relive each ephemeral moment. As with the faculty of make-believe in childhood, so, said Treves, every aspect of the show was real to him.

> ... the palace was the home of kings, the princess was of
> royal blood, the fairies were as undoubted as the children in
> the street, while the dishes at the banquet were of unquestion-
> able gold. He did not like to discuss it as a play, but rather as
> a vision of some actual world.

The life of the pantomime story thus for Joseph went on living, even though he was no longer there to witness it. 'I wonder what the prince did after we left?' he would ask Treves among a host of questions. Or, 'Do you think that poor man is still in the dungeon?'

There may well have been other visits to the theatre for Joseph, though no confirmation exists for those beyond an incidental remark contained in a later letter to *The Times* that Carr Gomm wrote after Joseph's death. But it seems unlikely that anything he saw subsequently could have matched the intensity of his first experience of living theatre.

24–5. The door and window to what was formerly Joseph Merrick's basement apartment in Bedstead Square at the London Hospital (*photograph by J. P. Entract*)

26. Merrick's specially built armchair (*photograph by Dr C. E. Taylor*)

Dear Miss Maturin

Many thanks indeed for the grouse, and the book, you so kindly sent me, the grouse were splendid I saw Mr Treves on Sunday He said I was to give his best respects to you with much Gratitude I am yours Truly
Joseph Merrick.
London Hospital
Whitechapel

Miss L Maturin
Sunderland House
Islay. N.B.

West Coast of Scotland

27–8. The only surviving example of Merrick's correspondence: a letter of thanks, with envelope, to Mrs Leila Maturin

29. Joseph Merrick, dressed in his 'Sunday best' for a portrait photograph (*London Hospital*)

30. The cardboard model of a church constructed by Merrick for Mrs Kendal (*London Hospital*)

31. Madge Kendal in Pinero's *The Hobby Horse*, a play in which she was starring at the time when she was using her influence on Merrick's behalf (*Theatre Museum, London*)

The Palace.

Couple from the Children's Ballet.

The Princess.

Cupid.

Jocelyn and Puss in Boots.

The Beautin Donkey.

Mdlle. Battona de Sortis.

Brother 'Eary.

Brother Williams.

Demon Lawyer.

The Princess's Pas de Fascination.

The Queen.

The King.

32. *Puss in Boots*, the Drury Lane pantomime seen by Merrick in 1887 (*from* The Illustrated London News)

33. The last known photograph, dating from 1888 when Merrick, at twenty-five, still had two years to live

34–5. The cast of Merrick's head and shoulders seen from two angles

36–7. The casts of Merrick's arms, and of one of his feet

38–9. Close-ups of Merrick's skull

40. A close-up of Merrick's pelvis showing his badly atrophied arthritic left hip-joint

41–2. Merrick's skeleton compared with the cast of his head

developed hip disease, which had left him permanently lame, so that he could only walk with a stick. He was thus denied all means of escape from his tormentors. As he told me later he could never run away. One other feature must be mentioned to emphasize his isolation from his kind. Although he was already repellent enough there arose from the fungous skin-growth with which he was almost covered a very sickening stench which was hard to tolerate. From the showman I learnt nothing about the Elephant Man, except that he was English, that his name was ~~Joseph~~ John Merrick and that he was 21 years of age.

As at the time of my discovery of the Elephant Man I was the Lecturer on Anatomy at the Medical College opposite I was anxious to examine him in detail and to prepare an account of his abnormalities. I therefore arranged with the showman that I should interview his strange exhibit in my room at the College. I became at once conscious of a difficulty. The Elephant Man could not show himself in the streets. He would have been mobbed by the crowd and seized by the police. He was, in fact, as secluded from the world as the Man with the Iron Mask. He had, however, a disguise, although it was almost as startling as he was himself. It consisted of a long black cloak which reached to the ground. Whence the cloak had been obtained I cannot imagine. I had only seen such a garment on the stage wrapped about the figure of a Venetian bravo. The recluse was provided with a pair of bag-like slippers in which to hide his deformed feet. On his head was a cap of a kind that never before was seen. It was black like the cloak, had a wide peak and the general outline of a yachting cap. As the circumference of Merrick's head was that of a man's waist, the size of this head gear may be imagined. From the attachment of the peak a grey flannel curtain hung in front of the face. In this mask was cut a wide horizontal slit through which the wearer could look out. This costume, worn by a bent man hobbling along with a stick, is probably the most remarkable and the most uncanny that has as yet been designed. I arranged that Merrick should cross the road in a cab and to insure his immediate admission to the College I gave him my card. This card was destined to play a critical part in Merrick's life.

I made a careful examination of my visitor the result of which I embodied in a paper*. I made little of the man himself. He was shy, confused, not a little frightened

* British Medical Journal. Dec. 1886 and April 1890.

and evidently much cowed. Moreover his speech was almost unintelligible. The great bony mass that projected from his mouth blurred his utterance and made the articulation of certain words impossible. He returned in a cab to the place of exhibition and I assumed that I had seen the last of him, especially as I found next day that the show had been forbidden by the police and that the shop was empty.

43. The 'deliberate mistake' in Treves's autograph manuscript of 'The Elephant Man': he scored out 'Joseph' and replaced it with 'John' (*courtesy Nicholas Reed*)

What Was the Matter with Joseph Merrick?

The question of the diagnosis of Joseph Merrick's puzzling condition was last left in the hands of the dermatologist Dr Henry Radcliffe Crocker (on pages 28–9), when, in 1885, he made his tentative yet positive suggestions to the meeting of the Pathological Society of London. Joseph was probably never aware of the fact that, three years further on, in 1888, he came to rest in a firm niche in medical history with the publication of Radcliffe Crocker's *magnum opus*, a two-volume work entitled *Diseases of the Skin: a Review of 15,000 Cases of Skin Disorder*. It was destined to be a classic among medical textbooks, and the second volume contained a section on the rare group of skin diseases known as the fibromas. It was here that he mentioned the Elephant Man.

> ·An extraordinary case of this kind was brought to the Pathological Society by Treves. I had an opportunity of examining the patient there, and at a show where he was exhibited as an 'elephant man'.

Like Tuckett, Bland-Sutton and Treves, Crocker had therefore made his pilgrimage to the freakshop in the Whitechapel Road. His technical description continued:

> The bulk of the disease was on the right side; there was enormous hypertrophy of the skin of the whole right arm, measuring twelve inches round the wrist and five inches round one of the fingers, a lax mass of pendulous skin, etc., depending from the right pectoral region. The right side of the face was enormously thickened, and in addition there were huge unsymmetrical exostoses on the forehead and the

occiput. There were also tumours affecting the right side of the gums and palate; on both legs, but chiefly the right, and over nearly the whole of the back and buttocks; the skin was immensely thickened, with irregular lobulated masses of confluent tumours, presenting the ordinary molluscous characters. The left arm and hand were small and well formed. The man was twenty-five years old, of stunted growth, and had a right talipes equinus, but was fairly intelligent. The disease was not perceived at birth, but began to develop when five years old, and had gradually increased since; it was, of course, ascribed to maternal fright during pregnancy.

Before saying what was the matter with Joseph Merrick, it is easier to say what it most positively was not. To begin with it was not the clinical condition usually labelled elephantiasis. The show name of 'The Elephant Man' that his managers chose has sometimes had the unfortunate effect of leading writers into a misdiagnosis and assuming elephantiasis was responsible. It is therefore the disease cited for Joseph Merrick in several apparently authoritative sources, but elephantiasis is a complaint caused by a parasitic hair-like worm that invades the body's lymphatic channels. It occurs only in tropical or sub-tropical regions, is transmitted to man through mosquito bites, and has entirely different features from those characteristic of Joseph's example.

Joseph himself was never in any doubt over the cause of his great misfortune. His distorted body must, he considered, be attributed directly to the frightening experience his mother suffered when making her way through the crowded streets at the time of Leicester's Humberstonegate Fair. As Bergen Evans comments in *The Natural History of Nonsense*:

> Once conception has been accomplished a further set of delusions obtain. Chief of these is the belief that certain impressions made on the mother during her pregnancy will affect the child. Of late years it has been held that pleasant impressions will have a beneficial effect and that the expectant mother should therefore keep herself cheerful, listen to good music, and frequent art galleries.

Beliefs in the imprinting of maternal impressions on unborn children are ever-present in folklore, from earliest times and in all cultures. The ancient Greeks advised pregnant women to gaze on statues of Castor and Pollux and other objects of great beauty so their children might be born fair and graceful. Similarly motivated, pregnant ladies in nineteenth-century Paris spent many hours in the Louvre, perambulating gently through the galleries. But as Mr Evans indicates, seeking for benign effects is only one aspect. Traditionally the avoidance of undesirable or even malevolent consequences needed to be taken into account at every step by women made vulnerable by pregnancy. Dr Károly Viski records in *Hungarian Peasant Customs*:

> The young woman must not hide a leaf in her bosom, because a similar mark will show on the child's breast; fruit should not fall on her, and if it does, she must not make a sudden move to catch it, as that will result in the mark of that fruit on the child. It is unwise to throw meat in the direction of the woman, especially liver, because in that case the child will get freckles.

In *East Anglian Folklore*, Enid Porter records how the eating of strawberries was and is believed in that area of Britain to cause a strawberry-coloured birthmark on a baby's body. In her *Cambridgeshire Customs and Folklore*, she cites the case of a Cambridge man born with his hands deformed, which his mother put down to a large, strange dog having leaped up shortly before his birth and pressed its paws to her stomach. Mentally retarded children born in East Anglia during the Second World War were often thought to be a consequence of mothers being frightened by bombing raids. In the Cambridgeshire fens, pregnant women traditionally tried to avoid the sight of a chimney sweep in case their babies were born black-skinned.

International folklore is rich in such material, and even in the most sophisticated urban environment the folklorist would not need to search far to find current examples. The conviction that a fear of spiders can be transmitted to an unborn child remains remarkably common, as does the belief that spilling a cup of tea or coffee over the mother's stomach may cause birthmarks. That modern medical science and Bergen Evans define such notions as nonsense matters little to those who believe in them. They may even be helpful to some mothers in modifying the emotional guilt unfortunately often present where a blemished or malformed baby comes into the world. In any case, it is only relatively recently that medical science has rejected these beliefs. Before that, over the centuries since Hippocrates, maternal impression was an integral part of a physician's advice to mothers-to-be.

In the sixteenth century a great French doctor of the Renaissance period, Ambroise Paré, listed maternal impression among the thirteen causes for the births of abnormal children. Two hundred years later in London, by contrast, William Hunter, who helped to raise obstetrics to a recognized branch of medicine, approached the belief more questioningly. He carefully cross-examined the expectant mothers who came under his care for details of emotional shocks suffered since conceiving. In no example did he come across a malformation or abnormality attributable to psychic injury. He did notice, though, that whenever a small foetal abnormality occurred, the mother would have little difficulty in searching her memory to find an incident to explain it.

But the rational William Hunter, in remaining sceptical of the theory of maternal impression, was well ahead of his time. The belief only lost ground during the nineteenth century as medicine began to find a more securely scientific and empirical base. It came to be pointed out that perfectly normal babies are often born to mothers who have been through appalling emotional crises; that, in any case, few mothers could hope to live through a gestation period of nine months without encountering some of the shocks normal to the business of living; and yet that most babies are born unmarked.

As research came to confirm, malformations of the foetus are generally present before the end of the third month in pregnancy while most events described by mothers happen during the later stages. Furthermore, no means could be discovered by which a nervous trauma might be transferred to the personality of the unborn child, for no nerve connections exist between mother and foetus, nor even an intermingling of bloodstreams.

More than at any other time in its history, the medical profession is aware today of the hazards that may damage a baby in the womb. It seems no more than common sense to advise an expectant mother to avoid certain drugs (including alcohol and tobacco) as well as serious emotional stress, and that any maternal infection should be referred to her doctor without delay. Thus, where medical science is concerned, the ancient theory of maternal impression, with its essentially magical linking of cause and effect, may safely be left to the attentions of folklorists.

At the time when Joseph Merrick was first examined, there were considerable problems of classification, and several factors made the situation even more perplexing. The first and most important source of confusion was the simple fact that the disorder from which Joseph has most generally been said to suffer was not then completely described or labelled. A second difficulty lay in its nature. It involved a condition capable of manifesting itself in many different ways, it being unlikely that any two cases, selected at random, would bear the slightest resemblance to one another in appearance or clinical history. A third factor lay in the extreme rarity of the disorder in its more striking forms.

From the vantage point of a century later, when we have a far wider if still incomplete understanding, the problem of diagnosis in the 1880s can be placed more precisely in context. It was rather as if Treves and his contemporaries were trying to comprehend the picture of a disease that had been broken up into a jigsaw puzzle, the pieces of which were widely scattered. No individual doctor was likely to find himself in possession of more than a couple of pieces of the jigsaw at any one time; he would be even less likely to know about other pieces of the puzzle, or to realize that the two or so pieces he held or knew about were related, let alone were fragments of a far larger as yet amorphous picture. That Treves, with the prompting of Radcliffe Crocker, succeeded in linking three major pieces of the puzzle and connecting the condition with the central nervous system was a credit to the high standard of British medicine in 1885. During most of the twentieth century, it has been broadly accepted that Joseph should be classified as a sufferer from neurofibromatosis, otherwise known as multiple neurofibromatosis or von Recklinghausen's disease. This diagnosis became controversial during the 1980s, though it retains its importance in the history of the medical understanding of Joseph Merrick's condition as new research leads into new areas.

Friedrich Daniel von Recklinghausen (1833–1910) was, as professor of pathology at the then newly founded University of Strasbourg, among Germany's most distinguished pathologists. He was a keen observer of disease processes, and was the first to describe several different conditions with which his name is linked. In 1882, two years before Joseph was exhibited before the Pathological Society of London, von Recklinghausen gave the first description of a hitherto unrecognized disorder. It was characterized by the presence of types of tumour called neurofibromas that were linked with the nerve trunks as well as by soft, lumpy tumours of the skin and areas of cutaneous pigmentation. He noted no other abnormality and suggested no cause for its origin.

Whether Treves or Radcliffe Crocker had come across von Recklinghausen's monograph at that stage of the story's unfolding is impossible to say, but even if they had done, it seems unlikely they could have linked the Elephant Man with the cases being described in Strasbourg, the manifestations in Joseph's example being so bizarre and gross. Indeed, it seems improbable that a diagnosis could have been confirmed even if Professor von Recklinghausen himself had been on hand to make a direct examination.

The name neurofibromatosis by which this disease is now known simply means that there is a tendency in patients who suffer from it towards the formation of one or more tumours of a particular type. The kind of tumour involved is known as a neurofibroma (one composed exclusively of a dense proliferation of nerve and fibrous tissue). Such tumours may occur singly or in great numbers within many different body tissues and can vary in size between that of a pin's head and an orange. It is the extreme variability in site, size and number of tumours that accounts for the variations of symptoms in individual patients. Despite their random nature it is even so the tendency to form neurofibromas that remains the consistent abnormality to be found in every patient in whom the disorder is diagnosed.

Most commonly the neurofibromas form within the layers of skin, and even here their appearance may be highly variable. In the disorder's mildest manifestations, there will be nothing to see but a degree of skin pigmentation, this taking the form of patches of skin colouring of a pale coffee shade. These may vary between mere dots and areas the width of a man's hand. Occasionally the pigmentation may occur as diffuse shading on one or both flanks. It is unusual to find a case of the disease in which such cutaneous discolorations are not present in one form or another.

A more severe manifestation of neurofibromatosis in the skin comes about when the fibromas form themselves into soft swellings. These may or may not be pendulous and they can vary between tiny warty prominences and swellings as large as a clenched fist. They are often present in large numbers on the trunk, but also, not uncommonly, develop on the face. Treves described such apparent tumours in great profusion in the notes he made on Joseph Merrick's disorder.

The most extreme skin changes of all occur when forms of diffuse tumour develop within the network of nerve fibres within the skin. These then become associated with a thickening of the skin and subcutaneous tissue, so that large folds of skin are formed; or there may be a diffuse enlargement of the subcutaneous tissues of a limb. Such a change as this most usually affects the flesh overlying the temple, cheek, upper lip or back of the neck.

It was dramatic illustrations of the disease of this kind that Dr Radcliffe Crocker and his mentor, Dr Tilbury Fox, were citing when they spoke of dermatolysis and pachydermatocoele (see earlier, page 29). In fact, this was the technical description that continued to be applied to Joseph Merrick's case over many years, for it was not realized that such cases might be explained as extreme manifestations of the milder forms of the syndrome described by von Recklinghausen. By 1909 the link had been assumed. In that year Dr Parkes Weber, a physician to the German Hospital in London and something of a connoisseur of rare diseases, wrote in an article on von Recklinghausen's disease for the *British Journal of Dermatology*: 'The most famous example of the class was undoubtedly the famous Elephant Man whom many must have seen when he was at The London Hospital.'

In the fatty subcutaneous tissues of the bodies of the more sorely afflicted, the neurofibromas develop as firm nodules on the trunks of the peripheral nerves and may be felt as tender, bead-like swellings in the limbs and on the sides of the neck. Wherever nervous tissue occurs in the body, neurofibromas are capable of forming, and they commonly crop up on the roots of the great nerves and within the skull or the actual spinal canal.

On the face of it, it seems curious that solid structures like the bones should ever become involved. It is therefore not surprising if this connection was one of the later pieces of the jigsaw to fall into place. Only at about the turn of the century did associated bone changes come to be recognized, as when, in 1901, Jonathan Hutchinson presented the case of a woman who suffered from involvement and overgrowth of the frontal bone of the skull linked with bony tumours. And, in 1906, Dr Cooper reported similar findings in a young girl. Such skeletal distortions were usually found to underlie diffuse types of skin tumour apparently similar to those Joseph exhibited.

It was not until as late as 1930 that Dr Parkes Weber put forward the suggestion that the bone malformations occurred as a result of the involvement in neurofibroma formation of the periosteum (the fibrous membrane that shapes and forms the surface layers of a bone). Once again Joseph Merrick was cited, Dr Weber remarking in his paper:

> The famous Elephant Man ... whom I once saw, and who died at The London Hospital at the age of twenty-seven years on April 11th, 1890, had many deformities of nature of pachydermatocoeles as well as many bony thickenings and outgrowths ... Irregular periosteal neurofibromatosis may well have played a part in his osseous deformities.

During the past sixty years, a number of other manifestations of neurofibromatosis have been recognized, and tumour manifestation has been described in practically every tissue and organ of the body. Changes have been found to take place in such varied sites as the intestines, internal glands, including the adrenals, the kidneys and the retina of the eye. It is quite possible that variants of the disease exist that are yet to be recognized. Meanwhile, varieties of neoplastic disorder have been categorized which bear close visual resemblances to the classic signs of neurofibromatosis but are clinically quite distinct.

But to possess any sort of unified picture of neurofibromatosis is still an exclusive privilege of the pathologist or medical scientist. From the viewpoint of the individual patient or a doctor in general practice the disorder presents a rather different aspect. To start with, it is not especially common. A doctor in general practice may expect to come across no more than two or three cases during the course of a working life. It is also important to stress that, in the vast majority of examples, the disorder is so minor as to cause little in the way of symptoms: perhaps a small, soft swelling that may be felt beneath the skin, or a few warty pimples hidden from sight beneath normal clothes or a patch of lightly pigmented skin. Thus the condition may often be ignored or never reach the attention of a medical practitioner. Cases suffering from disturbances severe enough to incommode them or threaten their well-being are considerable medical rarities and widely scattered.

The genetic defect responsible for neurofibromatosis turns up in a wide range of races and in virtually every corner of the world. Evidence for it may be present at birth or it may make its first appearance during early childhood, though relatively few patients come under active medical care during this period. In many instances, the disease does not progress, but remains static for year after year. Only in the most occasional patient will it metamorphose into a progressive form so that each year of life sees some fresh and tragic affliction. Quite early on in the study of neurofibromatosis it was recognized that it could run in families, often passing down through two, three or even four generations. In fact about half of all known cases have been found to inherit the disorder directly from an affected parent. In the other half of cases, it seems as though the disorder is sporadic and caused by a chance genetic mutation, no previous case being detectable in the family tree.

Perhaps the most comprehensive study of the genetics of neurofibromatosis was that made in the University of Michigan in the early 1950s by F. W. Crowe, W. J. Schull and J. F. Neel. Their findings, published in a monograph, *Multiple Neurofibromatosis*, cleared up many problems in understanding the inheritance of the condition. At the outset they evolved a clinical method for identifying individuals who had the disease in even its mildest forms. This was based on careful measurement and counting of areas of skin pigmentation, a method they called the 'six-spot test'. Its use enabled them to study the passage of the disease through many families.

Where the disease was obviously a familial complaint, they showed decisively that the disorder was inherited as a simple Mendelian dominant characteristic. In other words, in the families concerned the disease was invariably passed down from sufferer to sufferer without skipping a generation. Moreover, wherever such a sufferer from the disease became a parent, about half the children of the marriage showed symptoms and half were normal. The affected children were then liable to pass the disorder on yet again to the following generation in the same ratio, though children born normal could rest assured that their descendants would be clear.

One interesting point discovered by Crowe, Schull and Neel was that the disorder is not in practice transmitted as freely as might be expected. Many sufferers do not marry, and those who do seem to be relatively infertile. Sexual and general physical underdevelopment is certainly a recognized feature of the condition in a proportion of victims.

The Michigan doctors also threw some light on the origin of those sporadic cases that occur without any previous trace being present in their families. Such patients are also prone to avoid marriage, and, where they do marry, also prove comparatively infertile. Where, however, the research team managed to examine thirty-five children resulting from such marriages, they found that eighteen of them, or almost half, showed evidence of the disease. Obviously even in sporadic cases the disease may become inheritable.

There is at present no way of confirming decisively whether or not Joseph Carey Merrick was a sporadic case of neurofibromatosis caused by a chance genetic mutation. Neither is there any way of knowing in what way his mother, Mary Jane Merrick, or his sister, Marian Eliza, were crippled and whether their disabilities were consistent with the same disease. The only tentative inference to be drawn is that the fact of their being crippled provides circumstantial evidence for a defective gene perhaps being carried by Joseph's mother. Certainly there is no indication of the illness being present in any branch of his father's family.

From the moment he came under the care of the London Hospital, the Elephant Man posed an endlessly fascinating puzzle for the medical world. Alternative diagnoses for the cause of his deformities have been advanced from time to time, including the idea that he may have suffered from a condition known as Maffucci's syndrome, or that the rare disorder called polyostitic fibrous dysplasia could have been involved. None of these theses have stood up to the test of further investigation. In 1986, however, J. A. R. Tibbles and M. M. Cohen Jr, respectively Professor of Paediatrics and Professor of Oral Pathology and Paediatrics at Dalhousie University in Nova Scotia, published an article in the *British Medical Journal* entitled 'The Proteus Syndrome: the Elephant Man Diagnosed'. Named after the polymorphous or shape-shifting Greek god Proteus, this rare condition, involving a complex overgrowth of bodily tissues with bone distortion, was first observed in the late 1970s, and delineated in 1983. Tibbles and Cohen have asserted that there is 'no positive evidence that the Elephant Man suffered from neurofibromatosis; rather, there is good evidence that he did not and in fact had features that are fully compatible with Proteus syndrome'.

Former sufferers from Proteus syndrome, the aetiology of which is as yet unknown, were undoubtedly misdiagnosed in the past as neurofibromatosis victims. Whether this was so in the case of Joseph Merrick remains at present an open question. For the time being, as an alternative theory for his condition, the thesis of Tibbles and Cohen stands as a strong contender. They point out, for instance, that no authority who examined Merrick in life left a clinical note of the presence of the characteristic *café au lait* spots; though it seems rather a demanding expectation that the observers of the time might have singled these out amid his bewildering wilderness of symptoms. The current effect of their theory, however, is to place a qualifying question mark over the statements made firmly in generation after generation of classic medical textbooks – such works of basic authority as Kinnier Wilson's *Neurology*, Boyd's *Textbook of Pathology* and Russell Brain's *Diseases of the Nervous System* – to the effect that Joseph's case was a supreme example of multiple neurofibromatosis.

Meanwhile, in support of the neurofibromatosis thesis, Professor

Gordon Seward of the Royal London Hospital Medical College has defined six skeletal features that he feels to be consistent with neurofibromatosis. First there is the lack of symmetry in the skeleton, the bones on one side being abnormally enlarged while those on the other are more delicate and slender than could be considered normal. The superfluous outcrops of bone (exostoses) contain bone that has a coarsely trabeculated structure (the arrangement of the thin, internal supporting struts of bone) while the outer cortical bone adjacent to these is normal. The palate shows, on its right-hand side, a deep concave depression consistent with the site of a neurofibroma, later in part cut away at the Leicester Infirmary; and a corresponding concavity occurs on the antero-lateral surface of the right upper jaw. There are also widenings of certain holes, canals and grooves for nerves passing through the skull and lower jaw bone. These observations are all consistent with a diagnosis of neurofibromatosis within its range of variant effects and have been known and recorded in other cases.

The Proteus theory has been welcomed by a number of clinical neurologists for seeming to avoid a problem of identification with the Elephant Man among neurofibromatosis sufferers, this tendency towards identification being felt to represent a barrier in the effective counselling of victims of the disease. It is an undeniable fact that the story of Joseph's life continues to demonstrate an extraordinary power to disturb and obsess. On the other hand, present-day society continues to harbour immense problems with how it looks at those who are seriously deformed, whether through accident, disease or genetic mischance: it would often rather they did not bring themselves to its attention. In this we are possibly more, not less, hypocritical than the Victorians. The problem may be regarded as one of education, but education is no longer seen as offering easy solutions. The story of Joseph Merrick in this respect has the specific value of a natural morality on the theme of human dignity. Its most profound implications can only be where it touches on such questions, and it would surely be difficult to justify any retelling of the story that failed to do so. To be moved by it is to gain insight, maturity and understanding on behalf of our own sense of humanity; the implications are far wider than those relating to one clinical syndrome alone.

Recent major advances in genetics and the identification of individual genes in DNA samples from fossil as well as recent specimens mean that the present debate on Joseph Merrick's acute condition may eventually be resolved on a straightforward scientific basis. It is now in theory possible to check a sample of bone from his skeleton to see whether the defective gene responsible for neurofibromatosis is present or absent. Such a test still probably lies some way in the future. There are many pressing claims on the research facilities that are presently opening out fresh perspectives in the vital new area of genetic mapping and analysis.

We therefore cannot yet say that the disease from which Joseph suffered so drastically and dramatically has been fully and comprehensively classified. Whatever the diagnosis ultimately arrived at, we may be sure that he stands among its most sorely afflicted victims. It is probable that had Frederick Treves lived a century later he could have offered at least a measure of corrective and cosmetic surgery. In the context of his own lifetime he was largely powerless, despite his surgical skills. But there is a concise creed that doctors throughout the ages have attempted to follow: to cure sometimes; to relieve often; to comfort always. Frederick Treves was unable to cure or relieve Joseph Merrick's medical condition, though ultimately he did not fail his patient. It has become the social fashion to decry the philanthropic impulses so effectively put to work to secure Joseph's future at the London Hospital, but it is chastening to reflect on how society's attempts at the management of the acutely deprived and disabled in our own day might compare in terms of the inner degree of security and the individual standards of kindness Treves brought to bear in the case of Joseph Merrick.

Sir Frederick Ponsonby, a private secretary to Edward VII, classified Treves as a 'great surgeon, a man with a keen sense of humour but a certain contempt for the human race'. This was to ignore other facets of Treves's complex personality. In the case of Joseph Merrick he saw it as a point of firm moral principle that the rules must be broken, and he made it his business to do so.

CHAPTER II

The Burden Falls Away

Treves could only watch the progressive decline of Joseph Merrick with helpless concern. From time to time he would intrude upon Joseph to make further clinical examinations and chart the advances of the disease. The bony masses and the pendulous flaps of skin continued slowly to grow, and the stump in the upper jaw where the 'trunk' was formerly amputated at the Leicester Infirmary did not stay dormant but began to re-enlarge, forcing Joseph's mouth into new bizarre distortions. The intelligibility of his speech again deteriorated. He suffered bouts of bronchitis and the doctors knew his heart was no longer sound. They knew, too, that he must eventually succumb to his peculiarly fungating disorder, and assumed that the end, when it came, would be sharp and sudden, perhaps in the eruption of a violent pneumonia or following a rapid failing of the weakened heart.

There were further confrontations with the hospital photographer. The last of the photographs, probably taken in 1888, dramatically demonstrated the premature ageing effect for which the encroaching disease was responsible. In the space of the five years he had known him, Treves saw Joseph's appearance change from that of a youth to one of an elderly man. Having reached his late twenties he was entering into his old age.

Yet, despite the slow, relentless deterioration to which he was subjected, the Elephant Man seemed able to maintain an inner calm and contentment. The patient's days settled into a steady routine of reading, receiving friends, greeting those who passed in Bedstead Square. The daily baths and the ministrations of the nurses also punctuated the quiet hours he spent alone with his thoughts. His mind meanwhile turned more and more in the direction of religious questions, the devotional upbringing he had received from his mother beginning to reassert its influence. In this connection he welcomed the visits of the hospital chaplain, the Rev. Tristram Valentine, who naturally encouraged his questing into simple theology.

Mr Valentine suggested it would be perfectly possible for him to attend the hospital chapel services on Sundays, for he could sit unseen in the vestry yet still hear and take part in the service. Mr Valentine must have made something of a contrast with the Baptist ministers whom Joseph knew in his childhood, having a reputation for being rather a 'high' churchman, but Joseph sought his advice and instruction, and eventually asked to be prepared for confirmation into the Anglican Communion. Confirmation in the Church of England may only be performed by a bishop, and then only after the prelate has satisfied himself that the candidate is suitable by having undergone an examination on the catechism. If Joseph was to be confirmed, the services must be secured of a bishop willing to meet and confirm Joseph in a private ceremony at the London Hospital.

The bishopric of London was assisted at this time in its heavy diocesan responsibilities by the suffragan bishopric of Bedford, originally created by Henry VIII but fallen into disuse until its renewal in the 1870s. Dr William Walsham How, a country parson from Shropshire, had been appointed to the suffragan see, though Dr How was no routine parish priest. He took an essentially practical view of his commitments as a Christian, had a strong gift for the written and spoken word and was a scholar in natural history and biology. Several of his hymns are retained in the *English Hymnal*, including the processional, 'For All the Saints Who From Their Labours Rest'.

During his twenty-eight years as a priest in Shropshire he had declined offers of bishoprics in various parts of the British Empire, as well as certain comfortably upholstered livings at home. He had only been drawn to London through his conviction that there was work to be done among the deprived and often desperate lives of the people of the East End. He saw himself, in fact, as the East End's unofficial bishop, and worked tirelessly to raise funds for his poverty-stricken parishes by holding public meetings in the West End and the richer towns of southern England.

The London Hospital lay within one of his parishes, and he was associated with its work. He had already met Joseph Merrick, having been present in May 1887 to offer the blessing during the ceremonies at which the Prince and Princess of Wales opened the new Nurses Home and Medical College accommodation. When Mr Valentine approached the suffragan bishop with the problem of Joseph's confirmation, Dr How felt no reservations about suitability. In due time Joseph was confirmed during a quiet private ceremony conducted in the hospital chapel.

Towards the end of his essay, Treves mentioned one other aspiration that, he said, had 'stirred the depths' of Joseph's mind: the chance to visit the countryside to observe nature and experience it at first hand. He had read so much about it in books.

> The country as viewed from a wagon on a dusty high road [said Treves] was all the country he knew. He had never wandered among the fields nor followed the windings of a wood. He had never climbed to the brow of a breezy down. He had never gathered flowers in a meadow.

Dame Madge Kendal mentions that Lady Dorothy Nevill, who was one of Joseph's visitors as well as a benefactor of the London Hospital, offered Joseph 'a cottage on her estate for some weeks, on condition that he did not leave it till after dark'. Whether this conditional offer on the part of a descendant of Sir Robert Walpole was ever taken up we do not know. A similar offer by Lady Louisa Knightley was certainly accepted, and it took place, according to Treves, during the closing months of the Elephant Man's life.

Lady Knightley's private estate was Fawsley Park, situated near Northampton. Here Joseph could have the run of a cottage without restriction. The difficulties that always came into play the moment Joseph travelled, however, meant that arrangements needed to be especially elaborate. Treves describes how Joseph, in accustomed style, left the London Hospital concealed inside the depths of a carriage with its blinds drawn. At the main-line railway terminus a whole second-class railway carriage had been reserved for his use, run into the sidings so he could board it unobserved from the departure platform. Then, with blinds down, the carriage was shunted into the station to be attached to the main-line train.

At his destination the procedure was reversed, and once more safely concealed in a cab, Joseph was brought to Fawsley Park.

Considering so much had been achieved, with so much attention to detail, it was ironic that there should have been a breakdown of plans as he arrived at his destination. It was intended he should stay in a small cottage as guest of one of the estate workers and his wife, who would see to all his needs. Unfortunately the wife of the house was insufficiently prepared for her guest's appearance. As with other women who came face to face with Joseph unawares, the first glimpse was devastating. The moment she saw him being ushered into her home, the poor woman turned and, her apron over her head, fled to hide in the fields. When at last she calmed down, it remained obvious that she could not cope with looking after the Elephant Man. A gamekeeper's cottage lay close to the border of a small wood on the estate, and here Joseph was taken. The gamekeeper and his wife, people of more robust clay, greeted Joseph with kindness and offered their hospitality.

In his account Treves says that Merrick stayed at Fawsley for six weeks, enjoying the freedom of being able to wander unseen and unmolested about the woods as the estate was strictly preserved. Merrick wrote several times to Treves, and his letters overflowed with descriptions of the wonders he discovered, of the trout he watched darting beneath the surface of a stream, of the wild animals he saw, of the bird-calls he heard, of his developing friendship with an apparently fierce and noisy dog. The wild flowers fascinated him, and he picked and pressed them so that he might send them to Treves to examine. Treves privately identified them as the commonest of hedgerow plants, but valued them for all they represented. They enabled him to create in words an unforgettable image of Merrick 'who had once crouched terrified in the filthy shadows of a Mile End shop . . . now sitting in the sun, in a clearing among the trees, arranging a bunch of violets he had gathered'. It had all been, said Treves, 'the one supreme holiday of his life'.

Once again, however, the facts step forward to catch Treves out in poetic licence. Lady Louisa Knightley kept a diary. It survives in manuscript in the Northamptonshire Record Office. The earliest reference to Joseph it contains is dated Friday, 9 September 1887, when he was evidently staying in the family of William Goodman

Bird, a farmer at Haycock's Hill near the Northamptonshire village of Badby:

> Mother and I drove to Badby where two sad cases – poor old Powell dying of cancer in the face – and a young Billingham of consumption. Then on to Haycock's Hill where Joseph Merrick, the 'elephant man' about whom there has been so much in the papers, has been boarded out for some weeks with the Birds. I think it is impossible to imagine three more melancholy things – they haunt me; one can only pray – and remember that Jesus lived and died for them. Merrick has such nice brown eyes! I looked straight into them – but he is *very* awful to behold. Croquet with my darling afterwards.

There is another entry for that same year, on Saturday, 29 October:

> Wednesday I went again to see poor Merrick at Haycock's Hill and thence to Daventry to distribute prizes at a work show.

As a conscientious member of the upper classes, Lady Louisa Knightley struck a broadly equal balance between pursuing the social round and the performance of good works. The following year Joseph was staying at another farm in the same locality, adjoining the village of Byfield. On Wednesday, 19 September 1888, she recorded in her diary:

> Mother and I went to a pleasant enough garden party at Edgcott and I visited poor Merrick by the way – and found him very comfortable and the Goldby's quite reconciled to him.

The mention of the Goldbys seems to provide a reference to the unfortunate incident Treves describes. That Mrs Goldby was happily able to accept Joseph in the end is borne out by one brief entry for Thursday, 5 September 1889: 'Went on the way to see poor Merrick who is at the Redhill Farm again.'

Thus it was not one but three supreme holidays that Joseph Merrick enjoyed in the Northamptonshire countryside. Mr Goldby seems in fact to have been a gamekeeper, so Treves apparently reversed the households concerned. It is also hard to resist mischievously pointing out that violets were never in season at Joseph's holiday times. Redhill Farm nevertheless lay just about a quarter of a mile back along a track from Redhill Wood skirted by the main Daventry to Banbury road. Joseph could therefore easily have walked at leisure between the house and the woodland unobserved as Treves describes. Moreover he was, at Redhill, befriended by a local farm lad, Walter Steel, who told his family in later recollection how he would call on him each day to chat and pick up any letters he had written to take them to the post. He, too, was impressed by the interesting quality of Joseph's conversation and by someone he felt to be a well-educated man. Mr Merrick, he remembered, composed a great many letters, and would sit out of sight in the woods to write them. He also remembered that Joseph liked to read a great deal of poetry and spoke of the delight he took in the natural world.

Joseph was back at the London Hospital by 7 October that year, for on that date he dispatched a letter of gratitude to Mrs Maturin, the 'young and pretty widow' to whom Treves had introduced him in his memorable therapeutic experiment. Mrs Maturin had sent Joseph a book and a brace of grouse from her home on the isle of Islay, off the west coast of Scotland. The letter is the only one to have been rediscovered from among the many expressions of thanks Joseph must have written to his patrons during his time at the London Hospital. It is one of only two examples of his handwriting that are known to have survived.

If Joseph's body was degenerating as the decade of the 1880s drew to its close, his spirit somehow seemed immune to decay; his peace of mind and quiet contentment were evident to all who had contact with him. His life was growing more restricted, and he found it necessary to conserve his strength, making it his habit to remain in bed till midday. The afternoons he spent reading or writing letters. The evenings were the precious moment when he chose to escape from the confinement of his rooms to walk alone unseen in the hospital gardens.

His spirits remained good, and on Easter Sunday, 6 April 1890, he twice attended the chapel services, taking communion in the morning. On the following Thursday evening, he walked as usual in the garden, then retired to bed. On Friday morning, 11 April, he followed his usual custom, staying in bed till noon. When his nurse, Nurse Ireland of Blizzard Ward, came to attend his needs, she spoke to him but noticed nothing to cause anxiety. She left him sitting up in bed. At 1.30 p.m. a wardmaid arrived with lunch and left it for him to eat in his own time. And then, shortly after three o'clock, Mr Hodges, Treves's current house surgeon, came down to Bedstead Square to pay a routine call. He found the Elephant Man lying across his bed and saw at once that he was dead. The untouched lunch remained where the wardmaid left it.

The house surgeon felt so shaken that he thought it best to refrain from touching the body until he could obtain the help of a more senior colleague, Mr Ashe. The doctors had expected Joseph's end to be swift, but not so startlingly sudden. Only when Mr Ashe arrived was the body disturbed as the two surgeons examined Joseph together, turning him this way and that as they sought the explanation for his abrupt departure from life.

An inquest on Joseph Merrick was held at the London Hospital on Tuesday, 15 April 1890. Mr Wynne Baxter, the coroner for Central Middlesex, heard the evidence, and next morning *The Times* carried a full report headed 'Death of The Elephant Man'.

Charles Barnabas Merrick, hairdresser, tobacconist and umbrella repairer of Churchgate, Leicester, had journeyed south to perform the last unhappy service he could for his nephew: formally to identify his mortal remains. His uncle and aunt remained the only persons in his family to have stood by Joseph so far as was in their power, and he maintained contact with them. At some point during his later years he sent to Leicester a copy of *Robinson Crusoe: His Life and Adventures*, adapted from Daniel Defoe and handsomely illustrated with chromolithographs after watercolours by Carl Marr. The inscription on the flyleaf,

> John Ernest Merrick
> From his Cousin
> Joseph Merrick

is the second example of Joseph's handwriting known still to exist.

John Ernest, who was born in 1881, fourteen months after Joseph's departure from the household for the workhouse, was therefore only nine at the time of Joseph's death.

Of Joseph's father, Joseph Rockley, the bare fact was recorded that he was known to be still alive. Then the inquest moved on to its essential business. Mr Ashe confirmed the death had been natural.

> Witness believed that the exact cause of death was asphyxia, the back of his head being greatly deformed, and while the patient was taking a natural sleep the weight of the head overcame him, and so suffocated him.

Nurse Ireland and Mr Hodges respectively described Joseph's last hours and the finding of his body, and then the coroner summed up by saying:

> ... there could be no doubt that death was quite in accordance with the theory put forward by the doctor. The jury accepted this view and returned a verdict that death was due to suffocation from the weight of the head pressing upon the windpipe.

In parallel, on the same day, the house committee of the London Hospital used its Tuesday meeting to discuss the problems raised by Joseph's demise. Treves offered his comments to the committee, from which medical men were rigorously excluded, and the minutes were as brisk as ever.

> It was decided that the skeleton should be set up in the College Museum, a funeral service having been held in the chapel before the body was handed over to Mr Treves, the licensed anatomist of the college.
>
> Mr Carr Gomm read a letter he proposed sending to *The Times* re Merrick and Mr Carr Gomm was thanked for his kindness in writing it.

The point was that so much interest had been aroused by the Elephant Man's plight, and so many influential benefactors had stepped forward, that the news of Joseph's death was unavoidably a matter of public concern. Carr Gomm's letter was an attempt not only to offer the world a full picture of Joseph's life and death in the care of the London Hospital, but also to make account of his stewardship of the charity sought on Joseph's behalf. It was printed in *The Times* of Wednesday, 16 April 1890, immediately beneath the report of the inquest. Again it summarized at length the desperation of Joseph's life before chance brought about his admission to the London Hospital, and the generosity of the public response that enabled him to remain.

> There he received kindly visits from many, among them the highest in the land, and his life was not without various interests and diversions; he was a great reader and was well supplied with books; through the kindness of a lady, one of the brightest ornaments of the theatrical profession, he was taught basket making, and on more than one occasion he was taken to the play, which he witnessed from the seclusion of a private box.

The next paragraph made much of Joseph's virtues, of his confirmation by the bishop, of his attendance at chapel services, and how, during the last conversation he had with the chaplain, he 'expressed his feelings of deep gratitude for all that had been done for him here, and his acknowledgement of the mercy of God in bringing him to this place'. Then there was the six weeks' outing he had enjoyed at a country cottage 'each year'. Yet, declared Carr Gomm, despite 'all this indulgence' he remained 'quiet and unassuming, very grateful for all that was done for him, and conformed himself readily to the restrictions that were necessary'. Even into the very grave, Joseph Merrick's status as an infinitely deserving case needed to be repeatedly emphasized.

> I have given these details, thinking that those who sent money to me for his support would like to know how their charity was applied. Last Friday afternoon, though apparently in his usual health he quietly passed away in his sleep.
>
> I have left in my hands a small balance of the money which has been sent me from time to time for his support, and this I now propose, after paying certain gratuities, to hand over to the general funds of the hospital. This course, I believe, will be consonant with the wishes of the contributors.

It was the courtesy of *The Times* in inserting my letter in 1886, that procured for this afflicted man a comfortable protection during the last years of a previously wretched existence, and I desire to take this opportunity of thankfully acknowledging it.

Among those who took a personal interest in the news of Joseph's passing was Lady Louisa Knightley at Fawsley Park. She made a note in her journal:

I see in today's paper that poor Merrick, the 'Elephant Man', is dead, passed quietly away in his sleep. It is a merciful way of going out of what to him has been a very sad world, though he has received a great deal of kindness in it. Thank God – he was not unprepared. Now! he is safe and at rest.

When Carr Gomm's first appeal appeared, the *British Medical Journal* had followed it up with a report on the Elephant Man. Now, on 19 April, it did the same, its informant being Treves himself. The report reminded readers of the earlier reference and stated that Joseph's death had occurred at 'the age of 27, according to his relatives'. This at once created a problem since the article four years before said his age was twenty-seven then. 'His age must therefore have been overstated four years ago ...' The inquest report in *The Times* created further confusion by saying he was twenty-nine, but Treves was correct in accepting the relatives' statement for the *British Medical Journal*. Joseph's age at death was twenty-seven years and eight months.

He derived the name by which he was known [said the *British Medical Journal* report] from the proboscis-like projection of his nose and lips, together with the peculiar shape of his deformed forehead. His real name was John [*sic*] Merrick. He was victimized [*sic*] by showmen for a time; when shown in the Whitechapel Road, the police stopped the exhibition. He was afterwards exhibited in Belgium, where he was plundered of his savings. On one occasion a steamboat captain refused to take him as a passenger.

The report went on with an account of Joseph's appearance and deformities, and proceeded to 'say a few words on poor Merrick's last days and death':

> The bony masses and pendulous flaps of skin grew steadily. The outgrowths from the upper jaw and its integuments – the so-called trunk – increased so as to render his speech more and more difficult to understand. The most serious feature, however, in the patient's illness was the increasing size of the head, which ultimately caused his death. The head grew so heavy that at length he had great difficulty in holding it up. He slept in a sitting or crouching position, with his hands clasped over his legs, and his head on his knees. If he lay down flat the heavy head tended to fall back and produce a sense of suffocation.
>
> Nevertheless, the general health of the 'elephant man' was relatively good shortly before his death ... At 1.30 p.m. on Friday he was in bed (he seldom got up until the afternoon) and appeared to be perfectly well when the wardmaid brought him his dinner. Between 3 and 4 o'clock he was dead in his bed.
>
> Mr Treves, to whom we are indebted for the above details, is of the opinion that from the position in which the patient lay after death it would appear that the ponderous skull had fallen backwards and dislocated his neck.

A résumé of the inquest followed, and then in the penultimate paragraph there came a most interesting misstatement:

> We understand that the Committee of the London Hospital refused not only to permit a necropsy on the body of the 'elephant man', but also declined to allow his body to be preserved.

The fact of the matter was that, in the Anatomy Department of the Medical College of the London Hospital, casts had already been made of Joseph's body and the process of dissection was well under way. Unless this was a genuine misunderstanding, it is impossible to avoid the impression that Treves felt it would be unpolitic for the information to be made public. Perhaps he feared it might create distress for those who had responded so compassionately in contributing to Joseph's happiness and welfare as well as often cultivating his company.

When reading the various accounts of Joseph's end, it becomes clear that the doctors found some difficulty in explaining the eventual physical disaster that caused his death. There can be little doubt that Treves was the person most intimately acquainted with Joseph, and equally little doubt that he was one of the most gifted medical figures of his generation. It is probably therefore Treves's own account of Joseph's death in 'The Elephant Man' which should take precedence in so far as any version can be definitive:

> ... he was found dead in his bed ... in April, 1890. He was lying on his back as if asleep, and had evidently died suddenly and without a struggle, since not even the coverlet of the bed was disturbed. The method of his death was peculiar. So large and so heavy was his head that he could not sleep lying down. When he assumed the recumbent position the massive skull was inclined to drop backwards, with the result that he experienced no little distress. The attitude he was compelled to assume when he slept was very strange. He sat up in bed with his back supported by pillows, his knees were drawn up, and his arms clasped round his legs, while his head rested on the points of his bent knees.
>
> He often said to me that he wished he could lie down to sleep 'like other people'. I think on this last night [sic, since he died during the early afternoon] he must, with some determination, have made the experiment. The pillow was soft, and the head, when placed on it, must have fallen backwards and caused a dislocation of the neck. Thus it came about that his death was due to the desire that had dominated his life – the pathetic but hopeless desire to be 'like other people'.

The house surgeons, coroner and death certificate all spoke of asphyxia and suffocation; Treves, in his essay and the article in the *British Medical Journal*, spoke of dislocation of the neck. But Treves, it must be said, had the advantage of dissecting the body after death. He supervised the taking of the plaster casts of the head and limbs and the preservation of skin samples. To the frustration of future researchers, the skin samples were lost during the Second World War. The jars containing them dried out in the absence of staff who had been evacuated to Cambridge. Dry rot began to spread through the woodwork in the wake of the effects of bomb damage, and the rot affected the specimens. Consequently they were burnt when repairs began. The post mortem document was another casualty of the war. All the London Hospital's pre-1907 post mortem reports had been removed under the threat of the blitz to a 'safe' underground location, which subsequently received a direct hit from a high explosive bomb.

As Treves finally mounted the bones one by one into an entire skeleton, it must have been the conclusion to a gruesome and disturbing task, made doubly distasteful since this was for the surgeon the body of someone with whom he had been in a unique mixture of personal and professional relationship. Treves, however, was too fine a doctor to mistake the flesh for the man. Writing of their first encounter, he described Joseph as 'the most disgusting specimen of humanity' he ever saw. Towards the end of his account of the Elephant Man's life he sought to find words to express what he had learnt of Joseph's internal nobility.

> As a specimen of humanity, Merrick was ignoble and repulsive; but the spirit of Merrick, if it could be seen in the form of the living, would assume the figure of an upstanding and heroic man, smooth browed and clean of limb, and with eyes that flashed undaunted courage.

CHAPTER 12

The Figure in Time's Fabric

As is usually the case with those who, in any sphere of life, have no fear of breaking eggs to make omelettes, Frederick Treves possessed enemies as well as friends. Those who admired him did so unstintingly, but he also had his detractors among his medical colleagues. Some considered he had built his career on a certain rather unprofessional flair for publicity. He certainly possessed a notably happy knack for being in the right place at the right time. Even one of his more ardent admirers, Dr D. G. Halsted, stated in *Doctor in the Nineties* that Treves first became famous because of the care he lavished on the Elephant Man. It is only one step from such a statement to the innuendo that he used his association with Merrick for self-advancement and showmanship. 'The question is,' Tom Norman asked bluntly, 'who really exploited poor Joseph? I, the showman, got the abuse. Dr [*sic*] Treves, the eminent surgeon (who you must admit was also a showman, but on a rather higher social scale) received the publicity and praise.'

The shadow side of Treves's benevolence undoubtedly existed but was naturally never touched on by him or any spokesman for the London Hospital. As a part of the gratitude he owed, Joseph Merrick had needed to be ever-available for inspection by medical students and emininent scientists as well as shown off to visitors and Treves's friends and acquaintances. Tom Norman had heard a whisper that Joseph was far less happy with these circumstances and their dependence on charity than Treves ever implied or admitted. It even reached his ears that Joseph had sometimes asked, 'Why can't I go back to Mr Norman?' Joseph's omission in never divulging the fact of his mother and sister being crippled, his brother dead, may be put down to a suppression of painful memories for a complexity of reasons; but it may also in part represent a determination to preserve an area of privacy from the world, and even from Frederick Treves.

A milder accusation in circulation was that the hospital administrators had exploited Merrick as a publicity device in their fundraising campaigns. Meanwhile, in the streets outside, the people of the East End, mistrustful as always of the motives of authority, held for many years to the belief that the Elephant Man sold his body to the hospital in return for the care it offered him.

The public appeals made by the hospital on Joseph's behalf, and Carr Gomm's conscientious stewardship of the funds, make any business transaction involving the disposal of Joseph's body seem unnecessary and unlikely. As for the Elephant Man's publicity value to the hospital, it existed but was incidental. There is no evidence for any calculated or cynical exploitation in the dealings of the hospital and Frederick Treves with Joseph Merrick. To the question of whether Joseph's unexpected return to the scene in 1886 contributed to the growth of Treves's fame and fortune, however, the reply must be: very probably it did. Stephen Trombley, Treves's biographer, confirms the phenomenal extent to which the case of the Elephant Man placed him in the public eye.

The line of development being taken by Treves's career as a distinguished medical personality was well established by the time he first met the Elephant Man. The association is unlikely to have made much difference to his ultimate professional status, but in the context of Treves's need to build up his private Wimpole Street surgeon's practice (his surgical duties in the public wards of the London Hospital being unpaid), Joseph's reappearance could hardly have been more timely. It is hard to believe that the flurry of public interest in December 1886 did anything other than draw his name to the attention of the rich and influential and enhance the prosperity of his practice. It may even have been an important stepping stone in bringing him to the notice of the Prince and Princess of Wales.

In other words, it must have contributed a significant momentum to Treves's financial success, but only the most puritan moralist could blame him for unhesitatingly accepting his good fortune. The one valid question is whether his success in any way compromised his integrity as a surgeon, and that it did nothing of the kind is the decisive answer.

There is nothing to support any accusation that he deliberately set out to utilize his knowledge of Joseph Merrick's case for financial gain. At the outset he can hardly have foreseen the course events were to follow and his preliminary investigations amounted to no more than a diagnostic foray to try to elucidate a mystery. Thereafter his only writings on or presentation of the case were exclusively to professional colleagues or in medical journals. Not until the last year of his life, long after retirement from active practice, did he publish his recollections of Merrick for a more general audience in *The Elephant Man and Other Reminiscences*.

Even while Joseph was still alive, Treves was continuing to add corner-stones to his career in the shape of his medical writings. His third book, *Intestinal Obstruction: Its Varieties, with their Pathology, Diagnosis and Treatment*, based on the essay which won him the Jacksonian Prize of the Royal College of Surgeons in 1883, came from the press in 1884 and was swiftly regarded as a medical source book. The next year he produced *The Anatomy of the Intestinal Canal and Peritoneum*, based on his Hunterian Lectures. The book represented the high point of his achievement as a surgeon writer, becoming a classic of medical literature. In 1886, he edited a three-volume textbook of surgery with contributions from thirty-five leading surgeons of the day, *A Manual of Surgery by Various Authors*.

After that he seems for a time to have abandoned the pen to concentrate more on the scalpel. A young engineer was admitted to the London Hospital in December 1886, suffering from typhlitis, as appendicitis was then known. The generally prescribed treatment at the time was complete bed rest, with doses of opium to relieve the pain and enemas to relieve the bowels. The engineer recovered after six weeks, but it was known that the condition would inevitably recur and could next time be fatal. Treves was therefore consulted for suggestions of an alternative treatment, and he recommended surgery. It was a controversial and bold decision in so far as medical orthodoxy considered that acute typhlitis should simply be left to run its course.

When he opened up his patient Treves found the trouble lay in a kinking of the appendix trapping mucus and leading to inflammation. As Treves prepared to remove the appendix and freed the peritoneal folds (the layers of membrane that line the abdominal cavity), the appendix sprang back into its normal position. Treves therefore simply sewed his patient up again and the man duly recovered, though he was kept under anxious observation for nearly two months. There was no recurrence of typhlitis in the engineer, and, so far as is known, this was the first operation undertaken in Britain to treat chronic, relapsing appendicitis. It made Treves a leading authority in this particular branch of surgery.

Meanwhile Treves's reputation as a surgeon spread far and wide in fashionable circles. Sir Henry Irving consulted him when he inhaled the nozzle of a throat spray into his lung. He performed a desperate tracheotomy by the light of an oil lamp on the Victorian painter and president of the Royal Academy, Sir John Millais, who was a victim of throat cancer. Another rich patient, a Mr Fielden, donated £22,000 to the London Hospital in gratitude for what Treves had been able to do for him and the hospital built a complete isolation block on the strength of it. Mr Fielden then made further donations of £62,000 and left the hospital £100,000 in his will.

In the 1890s, Treves resumed his medical authorship, producing in 1891 a large two-volume textbook, *A Manual of Operative Surgery*, concerned solely with the practical aspects of treatment by operation. An abridged version followed a year later, and in 1895 his last full-length medical textbook, *A System of Surgery*, also in two volumes, was published. He was writing these during an intensely busy period as he continued to fulfil his duties as consulting surgeon to the London Hospital. He did not resign from his post there until 1898, the year after Queen Victoria's Diamond Jubilee celebrations.

A sequence of personal honours was now the inevitable corollary to the advances in his career. Following the outbreak of the Boer War in 1899, he saw service in South Africa as a surgeon to one of the field hospitals. He witnessed the relief of Ladysmith before a severe bout of dysentery laid him low. While he was still recovering, the Court Circular announced that Queen Victoria had been pleased to appoint Mr Treves as one of her surgeons-in-ordinary. Within a year the queen was dead and the Prince of Wales had succeeded to the throne as Edward VII. On 4 May 1901 the following announcement appeared in the Court Circular:

> Mr Frederick Treves was introduced to the King's presence when His Majesty conferred upon him the honour of Knighthood and invested him with the insignia of a Knight Commander of the Royal Victorian Order. Sir Frederick Treves who was Surgeon in Ordinary to her late Majesty Queen Victoria and is Surgeon in Ordinary to the Duke of Cornwall and York was recently appointed one of the honorary Sergeant Surgeons to the King.

Since the Royal Victorian Order is awarded personally by the monarch, and for services only to the sovereign and his or her family, it might have seemed that Treves was at the zenith of his ambitions. Yet only a year earlier a personal and ironic tragedy had struck at the family of this surgeon who was probably his country's leading expert in acute appendicitis. His younger daughter, Hetty, was struck down by the condition at the age of eighteen, and became mortally ill. He called in two eminent colleagues, but they could only gently tell him that if he could do nothing for her then no one in the country could do better. Her death cast a shadow over all the years that followed, though his most dramatic encounter with appendicitis was yet to follow. When Edward VII became ill almost on the eve of his coronation in June 1902, appendicitis was diagnosed. It was decided that an operation on the king's appendix was imperative if his life was to be saved and that the coronation must be postponed; it was Treves who stood by to make the historic cut and who drained the offending abscess, deciding it was not essential to remove the appendix itself. Twenty-one years later, in its obituary notice of the surgeon, *The Times* wrote:

> Though Treves had eminent colleagues who supported him, he was in principal charge and the real responsibility for the operation and postponing the Coronation rested wholly on his shoulders. Only a man of inflexible resolution, perfectly

convinced of the correctness of his diagnosis and proposed treatment, could have carried it through.

In Edward VII's Coronation Honours List, Treves was one of those who received a baronetcy.

It surprised many that this was the point when, apparently at the height of his powers, Treves chose virtually to bring his medical career to a close. But, he had once said, no surgeon should operate after the age of fifty. His was to be no idle retirement: he retained his royal appointments and became involved, among other things, as a founder member of the British Red Cross Society and in setting up the Radium Institute in London to pioneer the uses of radium in British medicine. The wealth he had accumulated, however, meant he had no further need to work for a living, while King Edward had granted him the use of Thatched House Lodge in Richmond Park as a home. There had always been about him something of a writer manqué, but it is hardly possible to build up a literary reputation by composing medical textbooks, however elegant their phrasing.

A book for the general market, *The Tale of a Field Hospital*, had in fact come out of a series of field dispatches he sent home to the *British Medical Journal* from the war in South Africa, and it had met an encouraging reception. Others were to follow. In 1905 he published *The Other Side of the Lantern*, an often vivid collection of travel impressions accumulated from a round-the-world trip. It was reprinted five times in the year of publication. The next year he brought out his volume on Dorset for the *Highways and Byways* counties series. For over seventy years, it has remained a classic of regional topography. To write it he visited every town, village, hamlet and manor house in the county by bicycle, pedalling a total distance of 2,200 miles.

The bonds Treves felt for his native Dorset remained strong throughout his life. He had continued to visit the county at every opportunity, and it reciprocated his interest by electing him first president of the Dorset Society. In 1905 he took a house in Dorchester, close to Max Gate, the home of Thomas Hardy, and while there he developed a former acquaintanceship with the poet and novelist into a close friendship. The desk Hardy used for his writing throughout his life was originally bought from Treves's father's shop in the county town.

Other travel books came from Treves's pen. A trip to the Caribbean produced *The Cradle of the Deep* (1908), and one to Africa resulted in *Uganda for a Holiday* (1909). A visit to the Holy Land produced *The Land That is Desolate* (1911), and then he undertook a close study of Robert Browning's long narrative poem in an Italian setting, 'The Ring and the Book'. This he described as: 'One of the finest, most imaginative and most human poems of the nineteenth century ... Some of the passages ... are amongst the most beautiful to be found in any country or any age.' He made an expedition to Italy to work out the topography of the poem, accumulating a profusion of maps, plans and photographs. The photographs he took himself (as he did for several of his other books), and was careful to take them not only in the places described by Browning, but at the right time of day and in the right season of the year. The result was eventually published as *The Country of 'The Ring and the Book'* (1913).

The outbreak of the First World War called a temporary halt to Sir Frederick's literary efforts and he returned to official duties. Only after the war was he able to move his household to Switzerland, to live on the shores of Lake Geneva and once again to take up his pen. Two more books were produced, *The Riviera on the Corniche Road* (1921) and *The Lake of Geneva* (1922). But his health was showing signs of giving way, and only one more book was to come. This was the title by which he was to be longest remembered: *The Elephant Man and Other Reminiscences* (1923). He was suffering by now from a weakened heart, but had recovered remarkably from a bout of severe pneumonia in 1922. In early December 1923, however, a sudden chill developed into peritonitis, and by the seventh of the month he was dead. His body was cremated at Lausanne.

The Society of Dorset Men arranged for Treves's ashes to be interred with appropriate ceremony in Dorchester cemetery, though a brief farce intervened when the customs refused to let the small container through unless they were shown the death certificate. Treves's publisher, Newman Flower, recorded in his book of memoirs, *Just As It Happened*, how he invoked the name of the king and obtained a special order from the Home Office to get the ashes past this bureaucratic obstacle.

The ceremony was in due course held with a most distinguished gathering, on a day of foul weather amid sheets of driving rain. After moving off from the house in which Treves was born, 8 Cornhill, the funeral procession moved on to St Peter's Church for a service, then arrived at Dorchester cemetery with its host of mourners. Lord Dawson of Penn represented the royal family; Newman Flower came for Lady Treves. Thomas Hardy himself had chosen the hymns for the funeral service, and determinedly went on to stand in the exposed cemetery, shaking with cold. As the rain poured down his face, the old man brushed aside the pleas of those who feared it would be his death. 'I have known Treves since he was young,' he told Newman Flower, 'and I am going through with it.'

Once he was alone in his study later that night, the great writer who had transformed his native Wessex into an immortal and peopled literary landscape by his novels and poems, confided to his journal the sparest of impressions:

> January 2. Attended Frederick Treves' funeral at St Peter's. Very wet day. Sad procession to the cemetery. Casket in a little white grave.

The experience of having known Treves, however, coalesced into 'In the Evening', a poem published in *The Times* two days later. Eventually, in its revised and polished version, it was included in *Human Shows, Far Phantasies* (1925), the penultimate volume of Hardy's verse and the last to be published during his lifetime.

In the Evening
IN MEMORIAM FREDERICI TREVES, 1853–1923
(Dorchester Cemetery, Jan. 2, 1924)

In the morning, when the world knew he was dead,
    He lay amid the dust and hoar
Of ages; and to a spirit attending said:
    'This chalky bed? –
I surely seem to have been here before?'

'O yes. You have been here. You knew the place,
  Substanced as you, long ere your call;
And if you cared to do so, you might trace
    In this grey space
Your being, and the being of men all.'

Thereto said he: 'Then why was I called away?
  I knew no trouble or discontent:
Why did I not prolong my ancient stay
    Herein for aye?'
The spirit shook its head, 'None knows: you went.

'And though, perhaps, Time did not sign to you
  The need to go, dream-vision sees
How Aesculapius' phantom hither flew,
    With Galen's, too,
And his of Cos – plague-proof Hippocrates,

'And beckoned you forth, whose skill had read as theirs,
  Maybe, had Science changed to spell
In their day, modern modes to stem despairs
    That mankind bears! . . .
Enough. You have returned. And all is well.'

The warmest tribute of all came from Queen Alexandra, the
Queen Mother. She sent a cross composed of flowers gathered in
her own garden at Sandringham, and with it a card bearing the
inscription:

> For my beloved Sir Frederick Treves, whom we all loved so
> dearly and now miss so sadly, from his affectionate Alexan-
> dra, Sandringham, Norfolk.

More than thirty years had passed since Joseph Merrick himself
found release from the burden of his earthly existence. It seems
odd, perhaps even significant, that Frederick Treves should have
turned back to the topic of the Elephant Man's life so close to the
end of his own. The first into print with a personal reminiscence of
the Elephant Man was in fact Sir Wilfred Grenfell, Treves's former
house surgeon, who included one paragraph on Merrick in his
autobiography, *A Labrador Doctor*. Since this came out in 1920

and Treves almost certainly read it, perhaps it had the effect of spurring him into thinking he should write down his own version.

After Treves's essay 'The Elephant Man' was published, others who had once had a personal acquaintanceship with or knowledge of Joseph Merrick included their reminiscences in various books, among them Sir John Bland-Sutton in *The Story of a Surgeon* (1930) and Madge Kendal in *Dame Madge Kendal by Herself* (1933). All of these to some degree leaned on Treves's essay to help with prompting their own recollections. The last to publish a first-hand memory was Dr D. G. Halsted, whose *Doctor in the Nineties* (1959) arrived in the bookshops when he was himself ninety-one.

In *Just As It Happened*, Newman Flower records an anecdote on how the surgeon author's last work came to be written. As his publisher at Cassell, Flower had pressed Treves to set down some of his medical reminiscences, and when he was shown some of the work in progress felt excitedly that here was potentially the finest of all his author's books. The manuscript included a magnificently written and dramatic account of the operation on Edward VII. Unfortunately, and quite by chance, Treves happened to mention the projected work to Cassell's medical director.

'My dear Treves,' he said at once, 'you can't do this. You can't write any reminiscences. It can't be done . . .'

To Newman Flower's frustration, he now found it impossible to shift from Treves's mind the idea that he might be inadvertently breaking proprieties concerning well-known people. The surgeon was adamant he could not continue. Eventually he said to Flower, to ease his disappointment:

'Tell you what I'll do. I'll write you another book . . . about the queer unknown patients I've had – patients from the great army of suffering men and women I've been mixed up with.'

As it turned out *The Elephant Man and Other Reminiscences* was a set of twelve anecdotal pieces, but pride of place among those of the 'great army' thus lifted out of anonymity went to the Elephant Man. It has already been said that Treves, as writer and narrator, continues to deserve our respect, that he was capable of working up a sombre, even morbid and subjective power in his imagery. An interesting example of this type of his writing occurs in the travel book, *The Other Side of the Lantern*, where he includes a thoroughly unscientific description of a mangrove swamp on Singapore:

> Dead creepers hang into the gloom of this forest morgue; dead boughs block every gap and path as with the debris of some grim disaster; about the ground are dead trunks, with shrunken and contorted limbs, and bare roots in worm-like bundles, that seem to be writhing out of the ooze.
>
> In the undergrowth of this swamp of despair are horrible fungi, bloated and sodden. Some are scarlet, some are spotted like snakes, some have the pallor of a corpse. All seem swollen with venom. There are ghastly weeds, too, lank, colourless, and sapless – the seedlings of a devil's garden . . .
>
> By silent and devious passages the soiled sea creeps into the swamp. It crawls in like a thief seeking to hide. When the tide is full the floor of the outcast wood is buried in fetid water; when the tide slinks out it leaves behind a reeking and evil mud, which is smeared over every bank and root like a poisonous ointment.
>
> To make complete the picture of this Slough of Despond one might fancy a hunted man in its most putrid hollow brushing the vermin from his wet rags and listening with terror to the tramp of eager feet about the margin of the mere.

There is a touch of melodrama in the imagery of 'The Elephant Man' which helps to make it so unforgettable, and it must be re-emphasized that the Elephant Man's story would probably remain unknown outside the specialist literature had Treves failed to set it down. Yet even up to the point where he submitted the manuscript to his publisher he continued to be haunted by second thoughts over the wisdom of placing this particular story before his readership. He wrote to Newman Flower:

> The story of the Elephant Man is, I suppose, unique and in the hands of a more competent writer would make very 'hot stuff' . . . I beg you to be absolutely candid about it. My books have done alright so far and I don't want to end up

with a failure. I read the MS through again before I sent it off and I am full of horrible doubts about it. If you say – and I am sure you will be Dorset straight about it – that it won't do I shall be almost relieved. It is no use to brag that every incident in the book is true; for I am doubtful if these are the kind of truths the public want.

Of all Treves's writings, 'The Elephant Man' is undoubtedly the one that will continue to be read long after the others are forgotten. If Treves owed Joseph Merrick a debt of sorts, he had gone far towards repaying it. In the air there is left hanging only one of the teasing, unanswerable questions of which history has many examples: had Frederick Treves not persisted in finding Mr Norman in the coffee-shop to get him to come and open up his freakshow on that autumn day of 1884, but had given up and returned to his duties in the hospital, would he ever have found himself standing at the bedside of Edward VII, poised to perform one of the most famous operations in the history of surgery?

Before leaving the subject of Treves's manuscript, it is interesting to note that when it surfaced for auction in Sotheby's London sale rooms in July 1980, it turned out to throw a small but significant ray of light on the long-standing mystery of how Treves came to deliver Joseph to posterity with the wrong Christian name. In fact, throughout 'The Elephant Man', Treves simply calls him 'Merrick', as he no doubt did when he knew him, in line with the social conventions of the day. Only once does he mention a Christian name, and this is where he states that among the sparse information he obtained from the showman was the fact that his name was 'John Merrick'. At this point in the manuscript, hand-written in a fine calligraphy unusual if not unique in a member of the medical profession, Treves originally wrote 'Joseph Merrick', then firmly crossed out 'Joseph' and corrected it to 'John'. The implication is unavoidable: Treves knew perfectly well that the Elephant Man's name was Joseph and that he had misnamed him earlier. He therefore corrected it to keep the record straight and had no reason to dream anyone would consider the matter further. There has been ample demonstration that Treves could be ruthless with the facts in the cause of telling a good yarn.

The publication of Treves's last book created wide ripples of interest. It was widely reviewed in the specialist as well as the general press, and the journal the *World's Fair*, a weekly publication devoted to news of interest to travelling showmen, carried an article on the Elephant Man culled from Treves's material. It was this that came to the attention of Tom Norman and stung him into writing a letter of injured pride in answer to the impression of him Treves had put forward. Tom Norman had been deeply wounded through his association with the Elephant Man. So far as Treves was concerned he was, he wrote, 'really at a loss to account for that man's antagonism towards me'. On one occasion he had tried to visit Joseph at the London Hospital, believing that the Elephant Man wished to see him, but had been turned away. He had retained a waxwork bust of the Elephant Man, commissioned from a firm called Meech in Lambeth Row, and featured it in his various waxwork exhibitions over the years. But though he might from time to time dispose of other exhibition stock, the Elephant Man bust would always be carefully returned to its crate and stored away. He never told any of his family why it was that this piece held such a special meaning for him.

In the manuscript notes he was putting together in his closing years, the Silver King created the self-portrait of a man of chirpy courage, who knew his faults, could acknowledge failures, but continued to face the world with unconquered enthusiasm and grew to be illustrious in his profession. His triumphs included the mounting, during the First World War, of a great show in Trafalgar Square, London, in aid of war charities, and he earned his place in the fairground histories. To protect and promote the interests of his fellow showmen, he helped to found the Van Dwellers' Association, which later became the Showmen's Guild.

In December 1927, Tom Norman wrote a letter to the *World's Fair* lamenting the passing of so many of the old showmen with each winter. His former associate George Hitchcock – the 'Little George' of his recollections – had died six years previously, having 'of late years been located at the Palace Fair Ground, New Brighton, but in former years he had travelled all over the country', reported the *World's Fair*. Tom Norman's days were also numbered and he was brought down by a throat tumour in the summer of

1930, on 24 August. He went out with a flourish, arguing good-naturedly with the surgeon over which of them was the better butcher. The ranks of the showmen, wrote the *Croydon Advertiser*, had lost a picturesque figure. The *World's Fair* was thwarted in its hopes of recording a grand showman's funeral. It had been, at his own wish, a quiet family occasion.

Of the other leading protagonists in the Elephant Man's story, Bishop Walsham How had died at the age of seventy-three during Queen Victoria's Diamond Jubilee year of 1897. As Bishop of Wakefield he had performed one last task of importance. A crisis was precipitated when Sir Arthur Sullivan declined to set the words the Poet Laureate, Alfred Austin, wrote specially for the Jubilee service of thanksgiving in St Paul's Cathedral, saying they were unworthy of his music. Bishop How was asked to step into the breach, and this he did, producing some alternative acceptable verses. The bishop who had confirmed Joseph Merrick at the London Hospital therefore also came to write Queen Victoria's Diamond Jubilee hymn:

> Thou has been mindful of Thine Own,
> And lo! we come confessing –
> 'Tis Thou has dowered our queenly throne
> With sixty years of blessing.

Seven weeks after the celebrations he died on holiday in western Ireland. His body was brought home to the Shropshire village of Whittington where he had once officiated as parish priest, and there, respected for his integrity and obstinacy of purpose, the great churchman was buried, his grave marked by a simple stone slab.

At the beginning of that same Jubilee year of 1897, at 28 Justice Street, Leicester, on 30 January, Joseph Merrick's father, Joseph Rockley Merrick, died at fifty-eight of chronic bronchitis. His death was registered, not by any member of his family, but by his next-door neighbour, Mr George Preston, who had been present at his passing. The address was the same as that where his twenty-four-year-old daughter Marian Eliza had died within a year of her elder brother on 19 March 1891, her death certificate stating the cause to have been 'myelitis convulsions', adding that she had no occupation, having been a cripple since birth. Joseph's uncle, Charles Barnabas Merrick, lived on in Leicester to achieve the ripe age of seventy-nine, dying there in 1925. His eldest son, Charles Henry, and his youngest surviving son, John Ernest, carried on with the family trade of hairdressing.

Sam Torr's daughter, Clara, who herself went on the halls, kept a diary in which she remembered how it had been at the Gaiety Palace of Varieties, Leicester, under her father's management.

> Everything was going lovely as we thought.
>
> We had a manager. He looked like a parson and knew about as much as one concerning the profession. We had several barmaids sometimes taking farthings for half-sovereigns.
>
> We had several waiters always missing when they were wanted. One would be on the top flat roof waiting for the pill man to set his stall out. Then he would throw a bag of flour down and upset all the pills. Another waiter would be fastening the ends of the coat sleeves of the other waiters so that they couldn't get their arms through. We also had a chairman which they played all kinds of jokes on . . .
>
> But the crash came, all too soon. One morning my dear Mother came to me in terrible distress saying, 'Clara, everything will be sold in a few days and we shall be homeless. Whatever will become of us?'
>
> 'Don't grieve so, mother dear. Something will turn up!'

And something usually did turn up for Sam Torr, who was another true professional and who, it is said, made and lost three fortunes during the course of his life, through a cheerful mixture of generosity and profligacy. His London career was, however, finished by 1899, his style of presentation being by then more or less out of fashion. He returned to Leicester, but injured himself falling from the stage in 1904 while attempting to perform 'On the Back of Daddy-O' in a state of intoxication. Briefly he became a publican, but sadly spent most of his declining years earning his bread and butter with a rather dubious turn performed in the back rooms of local hostelries. According to family recollection, he died quite gently in his own bed at the age of seventy-four, surrounded by those he loved. His end had come in 1923, the same year as Treves's death and the publication of 'The Elephant Man'.

Madge Kendal retired from the stage in 1908, but lived on

triumphantly as 'the matron of the British drama' until 1935, loaded down with honours and accolades, having received her DBE in 1926. She was, said Seymour Hicks, 'the very greatest of actresses'. 'No other English actress has such extraordinary skill,' wrote Ellen Terry, with whom Mrs Kendal was supposed to have enjoyed a life-long jealous rivalry, though like most such legends it was largely an invention of the press. On the other hand, Sir Cedric Hardwicke in *A Victorian in Orbit* had an altogether more waspish recollection of her. 'She was one of a raft of sturdy, stage widows,' he wrote, 'whose sheer, awesome vitality had enabled them to outdistance their husbands in billings and longevity.' Summoned to an audience with her after she had admired his creation of the role of King Magnus in Shaw's *The Apple Cart*, he found the encounter something of a trial, she making it clear 'that, in her view, the world had been running downhill since the death of dear Queen Victoria, accelerating with each year that passed'.

> From the number of pressing invitations to return to her house, which followed the first encounter, I could appreciate that she was in dire need of company – and I could understand why. She reminded me forcibly of Boadicea, that Amazonian English queen who mowed down Romans with her chariot wheels. Mrs Kendal was so terrifying that most contemporary members of our profession stayed clear in droves. Generally speaking, she regarded herself and her late husband as the last flowering of the dramatic arts.

Dr Reginald Tuckett, who first pressed Treves to go and view the Elephant Man, in 1893 went into a rural practice at Woodhouse Eaves, not far from the city of Leicester. He remained there as a general practitioner more than fifty years, well known for his strength of personality and independent viewpoint. He refused to co-operate with Lloyd George's and Winston Churchill's National Insurance Act of 1911 when it was introduced, and the advent of Britain's National Health Service after the Second World War seemed to him the last straw. He finally retired in protest in 1948 at eighty-nine, dying two years later, one of the last of the impressive breed of physicians who were the products of the great teaching hospitals of Victorian London.

*

In the quiet hall of the Medical College of the London Hospital, in a glass case tucked away among other anatomical specimens in their glass cases, the skeleton of the Elephant Man stands, apparently ready to face up to any casual scrutiny. His surviving memorabilia are about him: the huge 'pillar-box' hat Sam Roper had made for him and, at his feet, the cardboard model of the church he put together and presented to Mrs Kendal. The plaster casts of his head and limbs that were made *post mortem* are also there, and perhaps invoke something of the instinctive sense of shock and revulsion felt by so many when they first saw him. The skeleton itself, however, remains oddly touching, even moving, in its slightness of stature. The delicacy of the bones of the left arm still contrast strikingly with the random distortions of the bones on the opposite side of the body. The consequences of the old hip injury may still be detected, the severe atrophying of the hip joint being, in the view of Professor Seward, the probable result of tuberculosis setting in within the femoral head after trauma. The curvature of the spine that accompanied the advance of the disease is also evident. On the skull the effects are dramatic: the bone down the right side of the head looks as though it has in some way melted to a point where it ran like a flow of lava.

Bedstead Square has been swept away by successive improvement and modernization schemes at the London Hospital, but the room Joseph occupied in the basement still exists. Even this is not exactly as he knew it. There has been some reorganization of the internal walls and it is now used as a storeroom. Large asbestos-clad pipes from the hospital's central-heating system run around the walls, and it is impossible to conjure up any remaining shred of his presence. Perhaps it is only in the imagination that he retains an undoubted power to haunt us, though there has been a tradition among student nurses at the London Hospital that his ghost still walks the upper corridors where he was lodged after his admission.

Many of those who met and came to know Joseph Merrick were struck by his sensitive intelligence, by the sweetness of personality beneath the horrifying outer shell. If there were elements of naïvety, this was inevitable in someone forced by circumstance to live so much of the 'normal' side of life inside his head and to take his experience of sophisticated living from books and romantic novels.

Yet the lack of embitterment in his character had seemed a great puzzle, contrasting with the fierce cruelty of the attack fate launched on his physical body and the abrasive cruelties he experienced at the hands of men.

In his earlier book on Merrick, *The Elephant Man: A Study in Human Dignity*, Ashley Montagu included an important chapter that explored this apparent contradiction in terms of Professor John Bowlby's seminal work on the effects on personality of maternal deprivation and, conversely, the importance of maternal love to a child if it is to develop into a socially healthy human being. Unfortunately Professor Montagu had no choice except to draw his conclusions according to the face value of the information on Joseph's personal background that Frederick Treves happened to include in his essay. As the present book has shown, Treves succeeded in uncovering only the most fragmentary information about his patient's early life. The information on the period that he did include is also, for the most part, inaccurate or positively misleading.

Nevertheless Professor Montagu's final insights into the case match the facts as they emerge. He makes the point that if Merrick had really suffered the life of total deprivation Treves assumes, then the nature of his character would remain wholly inexplicable. From the descriptions of Joseph's character he deduces that he must have received a mother's loving care at least during the first few years of life, and that he must from time to time have later been shown a degree of supportive kindness by others. His mother's love, it so happens, was only withdrawn from him by her death when he was almost eleven, and after his father rejected him, his uncle, Charles Merrick, offered him the support it was in his power to give, while the showmen who managed his exhibition in England, despite Treves's description of them as vampires, showed a characteristic protective concern.

Certain so-called freaks have, in any case, demonstrated patience and good nature as integral parts of their characters. Perhaps there are at times other compensatory processes at work. Tom Norman certainly claimed that all the freaks with whom he had dealings were 'with but very few exceptions, as happy as the days are long, and were very contented with their lot in life'. At one time he included among his client showpieces the Scottish giantess, Mary Campbell,

... who used to sing 'Annie Laurie', and drank Scotch whisky and keep time with the next. But she was a dear old soul, good as gold. She lent me all her savings once, about £80, without asking, or a murmur. She was with me five years.

When William Hone interviewed M. Seurat, 'The Living Skeleton', in 1825 at the Chinese Saloon in Pall Mall, he found him neither unhappy nor miserable, despite the extreme emaciation of his frame. Seurat, in fact, had gone so far as to write a letter to the press to answer an expression of moral indignation about his being put on show at all. His present situation was, he said, 'more happy than I ever yet enjoyed during my whole life, and is entirely conformable to my desires'. He had hopes that the proceeds of his exhibition would shortly allow him to return to France to live out his life at ease. It turned out that poor Seurat was to die soon and leave his bones in London, where they went to join those of the Irish giant, Charles Byrne (also called O'Brien), and the Sicilian dwarf, Caroline Crachami, in the Hunterian Museum in the Royal College of Surgeons. With Seurat, however, it was the unembittered quality of his patience and gentleness that caught Hone's attention. These clearly have parallels in the later example of Joseph Merrick.

The story of the Elephant Man and the Victorian surgeon, Frederick Treves, who took over the management of his destiny when every other path was closed, never ceases to act as a sounding board for many resonances. So long as it continues to catch the imagination, then each generation will read into it its own mixtures of insight and prejudice. As with the relationship between Prospero and Caliban in Shakespeare's *The Tempest*, the emphases may seem to shift subtly in time as new social parables are read in or drawn out. The monstrous whelp Caliban begins to shade into the figure of the Noble Savage, an ambiguous representation of man in a state of sexual innocence. The omnipotent magician Prospero, who can control the elements and hence the lives of men, is revealed to have feet of clay and to carry responsibility for the things that go wrong as well as those that may be put right. Interestingly enough, the fact that Treves tended to see Merrick, if only subconsciously, as a late manifestation of the Noble Savage is given away here and there by a piece of phrasing, as when he describes Joseph as 'an elemental being, so primitive' or 'this primitive creature'. Is it possible that Treves was himself driven by that underlying sense of guilt the doctor so often feels when he becomes aware he must inevitably fail a certain patient over providing a cure?

It is perhaps one interpretation of the story to see Treves as a fundamentally exploiting figure sheltering behind an attitude of moral righteousness, while Merrick becomes the tame freak on whom society can safely lavish attention and so assuage its guilt at the vast inequalities of wealth created by the Industrial Revolution. This was a basis of interpretation Bernard Pomerance used for his distinctive play *The Elephant Man* that enjoyed much success in its productions on the Broadway and London stages. But interpretation implies a partial view of the facts, however valid or illuminating that view may be. The actual story of the Elephant Man remains constantly rich beyond the devices of fiction in its startling contrasts and turns of fate. The greatest presumption of all would be to think it possible to know or guess what it was truly like to have lived the life of Joseph Carey Merrick.

The closing and most valid image of Joseph to summon up is that of a squat figure, extraordinary in outline, limping without hurry in the starlight across Bedstead Square and into the gardens of the London Hospital. The freedom to walk there unobserved and take into his lungs the cool night air together with the scent of the spring flowers, became one with the hard-won freedom and dignity of his spirit under the stars: and so the limits to the span of his existence, the various griefs and injuries his life sustained, even the hideousness of his flesh, were transformed eventually into matters of small importance.

The Autobiography of Joseph Carey Merrick

I first saw the light on the 5th of August, 1860, I was born in Lee Street, Wharf Street, Leicester. The deformity which I am now exhibiting was caused by my mother being frightened by an Elephant; my mother was going along the street when a procession of Animals were passing by, there was a terrible crush of people to see them, and unfortunately she was pushed under the Elephant's feet, which frightened her very much; this occurring during a time of pregnancy was the cause of my deformity.

The measurement round my head is 36 inches, there is a large substance of flesh at the back as large as a breakfast cup, the other part in a manner of speaking is like hills and valleys, all lumped together, while the face is such a sight that no one could describe it. The right hand is almost the size and shape of an Elephant's foreleg, measuring 12 inches round the wrist and 5 inches round one of the fingers; the other hand and arm is no larger than that of a girl ten years of age, although it is well proportioned. My feet and legs are covered with thick lumpy skin, also my body, like that of an Elephant, and almost the same colour, in fact, no one would believe until they saw it, that such a thing could exist. It was not perceived much at birth, but began to develop itself when at the age of 5 years.

I went to school like other children until I was about 11 or 12 years of age, when the greatest misfortune of my life occurred, namely – the death of my mother, peace to her, she was a good mother to me; after she died my father broke up his home and went to lodgings; unfortunately for me he married his landlady; henceforth I never had one moment's comfort, she having children of her own, and I not being so handsome as they, together with my deformity, she was the means of making my life a perfect misery; lame and deformed as I was, I ran, or rather walked away from home two or three times, but suppose father had some spark of parental feeling left, so he induced me to return home again. The best friend I had in those days was my father's brother, Mr Merrick, Hair Dresser, Church Gate, Leicester.

When about 13 years old, nothing would satisfy my stepmother until she got me out to work; I obtained employment at Messrs Freeman's, Cigar Manufacturers, and worked there about two years, but my right hand got too heavy for making cigars, so I had to leave them.

I was sent about the town to see if I could procure work, but being lame and deformed no one would employ me; when I went home for my meals, my step-mother used to say I had not been to seek for work. I was taunted and sneered at so that I would not go home to my meals, and used to stay in the streets with an hungry belly rather than return for anything to eat, what few half-meals I did have, I was taunted with the remark – 'That's more than you have earned.'

Being unable to get employment my father got me a pedlar's license to hawk the town, but being deformed, people would not come to the door to buy my wares. In consequence of my ill luck my life was again made a misery to me, so that I again ran away and went hawking on my own account, but my deformity had grown to such an extent, so that I could not move about the town without having a crowd of people gather round me. I then went into the infirmary at Leicester, where I remained for two or three years, when I had to undergo an operation on my face, having three or four ounces of flesh cut away; so thought I, I'll get my living by being exhibited about the country. Knowing Mr Sam Torr, Gladstone Vaults, Wharf Street, Leicester, went in for Novelties, I wrote to him, he came to see me, and soon arranged matters, recommending me to Mr Ellis, Bee-hive Inn, Nottingham, from whom I received the greatest kindness and attention.

In making my first appearance before the public, who have treated me well – in fact I may say I am as comfortable now as I was uncomfortable before. I must now bid my kind readers adieu.

APPENDIX ONE

Was I so tall, could reach the pole,
  Or grasp the ocean with a span;
I would be measured by the soul,
  The mind's the standard of the man.

The Elephant Man,
amplified from an account published in the *British Medical Journal*

In November, 1886, a letter appeared in *The Times* from Mr Carr Gomm, chairman of the London Hospital, drawing attention to the sad case of Joseph Merrick. The letter attracted the notice of the charitable public, and through their very generous subscriptions the Hospital authorities were enabled to admit Merrick as a permanent inmate.

JOSEPH MERRICK is the subject of a very terrible congenital deformity, of so extreme a degree that he cannot venture into the streets, nor indeed into the garden of the Hospital. He cannot travel in any public conveyance nor mix with his fellow men. But for the kindness of his now numerous friends he would be cut off from all the common enjoyment of life.

Merrick is now about 27 years of age and was born of respectable parents in Leicester. Neither his father nor mother nor any of his relatives were in any way deformed. When quite a child his appearance was not sufficiently marked to attract any special attention, but by the time he had reached adult life the deformity of the face and limbs had attained to so extreme a degree that the unfortunate man was unable to follow any employment and physically prevented from learning any trade. His mother died when he was young, and his father, having married again, practically cast him off. There was nothing for him to do but to exhibit himself as a deformity in a penny show. Some features in the conformation of his head and limbs suggested the title of 'The Elephant Man', and as such Merrick was exhibited. He was dragged about from town to town and from fair to fair, and lived a life that was little better than a dismal slavery.

He was not treated with actual unkindness, but lived a life of almost solitary confinement, broken only when he appeared before a gaping and terrified audience as a hideous example of deformity.

Early in 1886 Mr Treves, one of the surgeons of the London Hospital, saw him as he was being exhibited in a room off the Whitechapel Road. The poor fellow was then crouching behind an old curtain endeavouring to warm himself over a brick which was heated by a gas jet. As soon as a sufficient number of pennies had been collected by the manager at the door, poor Merrick appeared in front of the curtain and exhibited himself in all his deformity. Merrick had a share in the proceeds of the exhibition, and by the exercise of great economy he had amassed nearly £50. The police, however, began to interfere and the exhibition was prohibited as against public decency. Unable to earn his livelihood by exhibiting himself any longer in England, he was persuaded to go over to Belgium, where he was taken in hand by an Austrian who acted as his manager. In Belgium, however, the exhibition was very soon prohibited by the police, and the miserable man and his manager were hunted from place to place. As soon as the Austrian saw that the exhibition was pretty well played out, he decamped with poor Merrick's very hardly saved capital of £50 and left him alone and absolutely destitute in a foreign country. Fortunately, however, he had something to pawn, by which he raised sufficient money to pay his passage back to England, for he felt that the only friend he had in the world was Mr Treves, of the London Hospital. He, therefore, though with much difficulty, made his way to London. At every station and landing place the curious crowd so thronged and dogged his steps that it was not an easy matter for him to get about. Indeed, at the quay great objections were raised to his being taken on board the steamer. When he reached the Hospital he had only the clothes in which he stood. For some time Merrick occupied a little ward in the attics, while every attempt was made to find him a permanent resting place. He had the greatest horror of the workhouse, and there seemed little to recommend the frequent suggestion that he should be placed in a blind asylum. The Royal Hospital for Incurables and the British Home for Incurables both declined to take him even if sufficient funds were forthcoming to pay for his maintenance for life. The subscription that was the result of Mr Carr Gomm's letter enabled the Hospital authorities to accept Merrick as a permanent resident. A room was built for him on the ground floor in a remote wing of the Institution. This room was comfortably furnished as a bedroom and sitting room, and to it was added a bathroom, for to Merrick a bath is not merely a luxury but, from the nature of his affliction, a daily necessity.

In this small room the elephant man spends his life, surrounded by innumerable tokens of the kindness of his friends. One of the first ladies to visit him, and certainly the first lady he had ever shaken hands with, was Mrs Maturin of Dublin. Mrs Kendal has been one of his kindest friends. She has supplied him with books, with pictures, with a musical box, and with numerous ornaments for his room, and had him taught basket-making as an amusement. He also owes to Mrs Kendal a very especial treat – a carefully planned and carefully disguised visit to a theatre.

Lady Knightley, in the summer of 1887, very kindly arranged a holiday for him, and with a little ingenuity Merrick found himself smuggled into a quiet cottage, in a remote part of the country far from the haunts of men, where he was made exceedingly happy.

The Hon. Mrs Gerald Wellesley became a frequent visitor, and gave him also a handsome musical box. Lady Dorothy Nevill presented him with a silver watch of which he is very properly proud. Among his other kind friends may be mentioned the Hon. Mrs Jeune, to whom he indirectly owes his country holiday.

The great event in Merrick's life was a visit from T.R.H. the Prince and Princess of Wales and the Duke of Cambridge, in 1887. The Princess was exceedingly gracious, and not only did she give Merrick some flowers (most piously preserved), but she also sent him her photograph with her autograph attached. At the following Christmas Merrick was delighted to receive from Her Royal Highness three Christmas cards, with a kind message in the Princess' hand-writing on the back of each. Of the royal visit, of the portrait of the Princess, and of her Christmas cards, Merrick is never weary of talking.

The following abstract of the Medical Aspects of the case is obtained from Mr Treves' account published in the Pathological Society's Transactions, Vol. xxxvi, p. 494.

The elephant man is short, and lame through old disease of the left hip-joint. The deformity concerns the integuments and the bones. The subcutaneous tissue is greatly increased in amount in certain regions, with the result that the integument is raised prominently above the surrounding skin. This tissue is very loose, so that it can be raised from the deeper parts in great folds. In the right pectoral region, at the posterior aspect of the right axilla, and over the back, the affected skin forms heavy and remarkable pendulous flaps.

The skin is also subject to papillomatous growths, represented in some parts, as in the right clavicular region, by a mere roughening of the integument. Over the right side of the chest, the front of the abdomen, the back of the neck, and the right popliteal space, the growth is small; on the other hand great masses of papillomata cover the back and the gluteal region. The eyelids, the ears, the entire left arm, nearly the whole of the front of the abdomen, the right and the left thigh, the left leg and the back of the right leg, are free from disease.

The deformities of the osseous system are yet more remarkable. The cranial bones are deformed and overgrown, so that the circumference of the patient's head equals that of his waist. This deformity is better shown by the engravings than by any verbal description. Bony exostoses spring from the frontal bone, the posterior part of the parietals, and the occipital. Irregular elevations lie between these bosses, and all these deformities are very unsymmetrical. The right superior maxillary bone is greatly and irregularly enlarged. The right side of the hard palate and the right upper teeth occupy a lower level than the corresponding parts of the left side. The nose is turned to the left and the lips are very prominent. The mouth cannot be shut.

All the bones of the right upper extremity, excepting the clavicle and scapula, and the bones of both feet, are enormously hypertrophied, without exostoses.

The patient prefers to sleep in a sitting posture with the head resting upon the knees.

The deformity is in no way allied to elephantiasis.

The following is added by Merrick himself.

'I should like to say a few words of thanks to all those that came forward with help and sympathy after my case was made known by Mr Carr Gomm in the public press. I have much to thank Mr Carr Gomm for, in letting me stay here, till something definite was done concerning me, as the London Hospital is not a place where patients are kept permanently, although the Committee have made arrangements for me to do so. I must also greatly thank the Hon. Mrs Wellesley, Mrs Kendal, and Lady Dorothy Nevill who have been very kind to me, and lastly my kind doctor, Mr Treves, whose visits I greatly prize, as many more in the hospital do, besides me. He is both friend and doctor to me. I have a nice bright room, made cheerful with flowers, books, and pictures. I am very comfortable, and I may say as happy as my condition will allow me to be.

> '"'Tis true my form is something odd,
> But blaming me is blaming God;
> Could I create myself anew
> I would not fail in pleasing you.
>
> '"If I could reach from pole to pole
> Or grasp the ocean with a span,
> I would be measured by the soul;
> The mind's the standard of the man."'

'The Elephant Man' by Sir Frederick Treves

In the Mile End Road, opposite to the London Hospital, there was (and possibly still is) a line of small shops. Among them was a vacant greengrocer's which was to let. The whole of the front of the shop, with the exception of the door, was hidden by a hanging sheet of canvas on which was the announcement that the Elephant Man was to be seen within and that the price of admission was twopence. Painted on the canvas in primitive colours was a life-size portrait of the Elephant Man. This very crude production depicted a frightful creature that could only have been possible in a nightmare. It was the figure of a man with the characteristics of an elephant. The transfiguration was not far advanced. There was still more of the man than of the beast. This fact – that it was still human – was the most repellent attribute of the creature. There was nothing about it of the pitiableness of the misshapened or the deformed, nothing of the grotesqueness of the freak, but merely the loathing insinuation of a man being changed into an animal. Some palm trees in the background of the picture suggested a jungle and might have led the imaginative to assume that it was in this wild that the perverted object had roamed.

When I first became aware of this phenomenon the exhibition was closed, but a well-informed boy sought the proprietor in a public house and I was granted a private view on payment of a shilling. The shop was empty and grey with dust. Some old tins and a few shrivelled potatoes occupied a shelf and some vague, vegetable refuse the window. The light in the place was dim, being obscured by the painted placard outside. The far end of the shop – where I expect the late proprietor sat at a desk – was cut off by a curtain or rather by a red tablecloth suspended from a cord by a few rings. The room was cold and dank, for it was the month of November. The year, I might say, was 1884.

The showman pulled back the curtain and revealed a bent figure crouching on a stool and covered by a brown blanket. In front of it, on a tripod, was a large brick heated by a Bunsen burner. Over this the creature was huddled to warm itself. It never moved when the curtain was drawn back. Locked up in an empty shop and lit by the faint blue light of the gas jet, this hunched-up figure was the embodiment of loneliness. It might have been a captive in a cavern or a wizard watching for unholy manifestations in the ghostly flame. Outside the sun was shining and one could hear the footsteps of the passers-by, a tune whistled by a boy and the commonplace hum of traffic in the road.

The showman – speaking as if to a dog – called out harshly: 'Stand up!' The thing arose slowly and let the blanket that covered its head and back fall to the ground. There stood revealed the most disgusting specimen of humanity that I have ever seen. In the course of my profession I had come upon lamentable deformities of the face due to injury or disease, as well as mutilations and contortions of the body depending upon like causes; but at no time had I met with such a degraded or perverted version of a human being as this lone figure displayed. He was naked to the waist, his feet were bare, he wore a pair of threadbare trousers that had once belonged to some fat gentleman's dress suit.

From the intensified painting in the street I had imagined the Elephant Man to be of gigantic size. This, however, was a little man below the average height and made to look shorter by the bowing of his back. The most striking feature about him was the enormous and misshapened head. From the brow there projected a huge bony mass like a loaf, while from the back of the head hung a bag of spongy, fungous-looking skin, the surface of which was comparable to brown cauliflower. On the top of the skull were a few long lank hairs. The osseous growth on the forehead almost occluded one eye. The circumference of the head was no less than that of the man's waist. From the upper jaw there projected another mass of bone. It protruded from the mouth like a pink stump, turning the upper lip inside out and making the mouth a mere slobbering aperture. This growth from the jaw had been so exaggerated in the painting as to appear to be a rudimentary trunk or tusk. The nose was merely a lump of flesh, only recognizable as a nose from its position. The face was no more capable of expression than a block of gnarled wood. The back was horrible, because from it hung, as far down as the middle of the thigh, huge, sack-like masses of flesh covered by the same loathsome cauliflower skin.

The right arm was of enormous size and shapeless. It suggested the limb of the subject of elephantiasis. It was overgrown also with pendent masses of the same cauliflower-like skin. The hand was large and clumsy – a fin or paddle rather than a hand. There was no distinction between the palm and the back. The thumb had the appearance of a radish, while the fingers might have been thick, tuberous roots. As a limb it was almost useless. The other arm was remarkable by contrast. It was not only normal but was, moreover, a delicately shaped limb covered with fine skin and provided with a beautiful hand which any woman might have envied. From the chest hung a bag of the same repulsive flesh. It was like a dewlap suspended from the neck of a lizard. The lower limbs had the characters of the deformed arm. They were unwieldy, dropsical looking and grossly misshapened.

To add a further burden to his trouble the wretched man, when a boy, developed hip disease, which had left him permanently lame, so that he could only walk with a stick. He was thus denied all means of escape from his tormentors. As he told me later, he could never run away. One other feature must be mentioned to emphasize his isolation from his kind. Although he was already repellent enough, there arose from the fungous skin-growth with which he was almost covered a very sickening stench which was hard to tolerate. From the showman I learnt nothing about the Elephant Man, except that he was English, that his name was John Merrick and that he was twenty-one years of age.

As at the time of my discovery of the Elephant Man I was the Lecturer on Anatomy at the Medical College opposite, I was anxious to examine him in detail and to prepare an account of his abnormalities. I therefore arranged with the showman that I should interview his strange exhibit in my room at the college. I became at once conscious of a difficulty. The Elephant Man could not show himself in the streets. He would have been mobbed by the crowd and seized by the police. He was, in fact, as secluded from the world as the Man with the Iron Mask. He had, however, a disguise, although it was almost as startling as he was himself. It consisted of a long black cloak which reached to the ground. Whence the cloak had been obtained I cannot imagine. I had only seen such a garment on the stage wrapped about the figure of a Venetian bravo. The recluse was provided with a pair of bag-like slippers in which to hide his deformed feet. On his head was a cap of a kind that never before was seen. It was black like the cloak, had a wide peak, and the general outline of a yachting cap. As the circumference of Merrick's head was that of a man's waist, the size of this head-gear may be imagined. From the attachment of the peak a grey flannel curtain hung in front of the face. In this mask was cut a wide horizontal slit through which the wearer could look out. This costume, worn by a bent man hobbling along with a stick, is probably the most remarkable and the most uncanny that has as yet been designed. I arranged that Merrick should cross the road in a cab, and to insure his immediate admission to the college I gave him my card. This card was destined to play a critical part in Merrick's life.

I made a careful examination of my visitor the result of which I embodied in a paper.[1] I made little of the man himself. He was shy, confused, not a little frightened and evidently much cowed. Moreover, his speech was almost unintelligible. The great bony mass that projected from his mouth blurred his utterance and made the articulation of certain words impossible. He returned in a cab to the place of exhibition, and I assumed that I had seen the last of him, especially as I found next day that the show had been forbidden by the police and that the shop was empty.

I supposed that Merrick was imbecile and had been imbecile from birth. The fact that his face was incapable of expression, that his speech was a mere spluttering and his attitude that of one whose mind was void of all emotions and concerns gave grounds for this belief. The conviction was no doubt encouraged by the hope that his intellect was the blank I imagined it to be. That he

1 *British Medical Journal*, Dec. 1886, and April 1890

could appreciate his position was unthinkable. Here was a man in the heyday of youth who was so vilely deformed that everyone he met confronted him with a look of horror and disgust. He was taken about the country to be exhibited as a monstrosity and an object of loathing. He was shunned like a leper, housed like a wild beast, and got his only view of the world from a peephole in a showman's cart. He was, moreover, lame, had but one available arm, and could hardly make his utterances understood. It was not until I came to know that Merrick was highly intelligent, that he possessed an acute sensibility and – worse than all – a romantic imagination that I realized the overwhelming tragedy of his life.

The episode of the Elephant Man was, I imagined, closed; but I was fated to meet him again – two years later – under more dramatic conditions. In England the showman and Merrick had been moved on from place to place by the police, who considered the exhibition degrading and among the things that could not be allowed. It was hoped that in the uncritical retreats of Mile End a more abiding peace would be found. But it was not to be. The official mind there, as elsewhere, very properly decreed that the public exposure of Merrick and his deformities transgressed the limits of decency. The show must close.

The showman, in despair, fled with his charge to the Continent. Whither he roamed at first I do not know; but he came finally to Brussels. His reception was discouraging. Brussels was firm; the exhibition was banned; it was brutal, indecent and immoral, and could not be permitted within the confines of Belgium. Merrick was thus no longer of value. He was no longer a source of profitable entertainment. He was a burden. He must be got rid of. The elimination of Merrick was a simple matter. He could offer no resistance. He was as docile as a sick sheep. The impresario, having robbed Merrick of his paltry savings, gave him a ticket to London, saw him into the train and no doubt in parting condemned him to perdition.

His destination was Liverpool Street. The journey may be imagined. Merrick was in his alarming outdoor garb. He would be harried by an eager mob as he hobbled along the quay. They would run ahead to get a look at him. They would lift the hem of his cloak to peep at his body. He would try to hide in the train or in some dark corner of the boat, but never could he be free from that ring of curious eyes or from those whispers of fright and aversion. He had but a few shillings in his pocket and nothing either to eat or drink on the way. A panic-dazed dog with a label on his collar would have received some sympathy and possibly some kindness. Merrick received none.

What was he to do when he reached London? He had not a friend in the world. He knew no more of London than he knew of Pekin. How could he find a lodging, or what lodging-house keeper would dream of taking him in? All he wanted was to hide. What most he dreaded were the open street and the gaze of his fellow-men. If even he crept into a cellar the horrid eyes and the still more dreaded whispers would follow him to its depths. Was there ever such a home-coming!

At Liverpool Street he was rescued from the crowd by the police and taken into the third-class waiting-room. Here he sank on the floor in the darkest corner. The police were at a loss what to do with him. They had dealt with strange and mouldy tramps, but never with such an object as this. He could not explain himself. His speech was so maimed that he might as well have spoken in Arabic. He had, however, something with him which he produced with a ray of hope. It was my card.

The card simplified matters. It made it evident that this curious creature had an acquaintance and that the individual must be sent for. A messenger was dispatched to the London Hospital which is comparatively near at hand. Fortunately I was in the building and returned at once with the messenger to the station. In the waiting-room I had some difficulty in making a way through the crowd, but there, on the floor in the corner, was Merrick. He looked a mere heap. It seemed as if he had been thrown there like a bundle. He was so huddled up and so helpless looking that he might have had both his arms and his legs broken. He seemed pleased to see me, but he was nearly done. The journey and want of food had reduced him to the last stage of exhaustion. The police kindly helped him into a cab, and I drove him at once to the hospital. He appeared to be content, for he fell asleep almost as soon as he was seated and slept to the journey's end. He never said a word, but seemed to be satisfied that all was well.

In the attics of the hospital was an isolation ward with a single bed. It was used for emergency purposes – for a case of delirium tremens, for a man who had become suddenly insane or for a patient with an undetermined fever. Here the Elephant Man was deposited on a bed, was made comfortable and was supplied with food. I had been guilty of an irregularity in admitting such a case, for the hospital was neither a refuge nor a home for incurables. Chronic cases were not accepted, but only those requiring active treatment, and Merrick was not in need of such treatment. I applied to the sympathetic chairman of the committee, Mr Carr Gomm, who not only was good enough to approve my action but who agreed with me that Merrick must not again be turned out into the world.

Mr Carr Gomm wrote a letter to *The Times* detailing the circumstances of the refugee and asking for money for his support. So generous is the English public that in a few days – I think in a week – enough money was forthcoming to maintain Merrick for life without any charge upon the hospital funds. There chanced to be two empty rooms at the back of the hospital which were little used. They were on the ground floor, were out of the way, and opened upon a large courtyard called Bedstead Square, because here the iron beds were marshalled for cleaning and painting. The front room was converted into a bed-sitting room and the smaller chamber into a bathroom. The condition of Merrick's skin rendered a bath at least once a day a necessity, and I might here mention that with the use of the bath the unpleasant odour to which I have referred ceased to be noticeable. Merrick took up his abode in the hospital in December, 1886.

Merrick had now something he had never dreamed of, never supposed to be possible – a home of his own for life. I at once began to make myself acquainted with him to endeavour to understand his mentality. It was a study of much interest. I very soon learnt his speech so that I could talk freely with him. This afforded him great satisfaction, for, curiously enough, he had a passion for conversation, yet all his life had had no one to talk to. I – having then much leisure – saw him almost every day, and made a point of spending some two hours with him every Sunday morning when he would chatter almost without ceasing. It was unreasonable to èxpect one nurse to attend to him continuously, but there was no lack of temporary volunteers. As they did not all acquire his speech it came about that I had occasionally to act as an interpreter.

I found Merrick, as I have said, remarkably intelligent. He had learnt to read and had become a most voracious reader. I think he had been taught when he was in hospital with his diseased hip. His range of books was limited. The Bible and Prayer Book he knew intimately, but he had subsisted for the most part upon newspapers, or rather upon such fragments of old journals as he had chanced to pick up. He had read a few stories and some elementary lesson books, but the delight of his life was a romance, especially a love romance. These tales were very real to him, as real as any narrative in the Bible, so that he would tell them to me as incidents in the lives of people who had lived. In his outlook upon the world he was a child, yet a child with some of the tempestuous feelings of a man. He was an elemental being, so primitive that he might have spent the twenty-three years of his life immured in a cave.

Of his early days I could learn but little. He was very loath to talk about the past. It was a nightmare, the shudder of which was still upon him. He was born, he believed, in or about Leicester. Of his father he knew absolutely nothing. Of his mother he had some memory. It was very faint and had, I think, been elaborated in his mind into something definite. Mothers figured in the tales he had read, and he wanted his mother to be one of those comfortable lullaby-singing persons who are so lovable. In his subconscious mind there was apparently a germ of recollection in which someone figured who had been kind to him. He clung to this conception and made it more real by invention, for since the day when he could toddle no one had been kind to him. As an infant he must have been repellent, although his deformities did not become gross until he had attained his full stature.

It was a favourite belief of his that his mother was beautiful. The fiction was, I am aware, one of his own making, but it was a great joy to him. His mother, lovely as she may have been, basely deserted him when he was very small, so small that his earliest clear memories were of the workhouse to which he had been taken. Worthless and inhuman as this mother was, he spoke of her with pride and even with reverence. Once, when referring to his own appearance, he said: 'It *is* very strange, for, you see, mother was so beautiful.'

The rest of Merrick's life up to the time that I met him at Liverpool Street Station was one dull record of degradation and squalor. He was dragged from town to town and from fair to fair as if he were a strange beast in a cage. A dozen times a day he would have to expose his nakedness and his piteous deformities before a gaping crowd who greeted him with such mutterings as 'Oh! what a horror! What a beast!' He had had no childhood. He had had no boyhood. He had never experienced pleasure. He knew nothing of the joy of living nor of the fun of things. His sole idea of happiness was to creep into the dark and hide. Shut up alone in a booth, awaiting the next exhibition, how mocking must have sounded the laughter and merriment of the boys and girls outside who were enjoying the 'fun of the fair'! He had no past to look back upon and no future to look forward to. At the age of twenty he was a creature without hope. There was nothing in front of him but a vista of caravans creeping along a road, of rows of glaring show tents and of circles of staring eyes with, at the end, the spectacle of a broken man in a poor law infirmary.

Those who are interested in the evolution of character might speculate as to the effect of this brutish life upon a sensitive and intelligent man. It would be reasonable to surmise that he would become a spiteful and malignant misanthrope, swollen with venom and filled with hatred of his fellow-men, or, on the other hand, that he would degenerate into a despairing melancholic on the verge of idiocy. Merrick, however, was no such being. He had passed through the fire and had come out unscathed. His troubles had ennobled him. He showed himself to be a gentle, affectionate and lovable creature, as amiable as a happy woman, free from any trace of cynicism or resentment, without a grievance and without an unkind word for anyone. I have never heard him complain. I have never heard him deplore his ruined life or resent the treatment he had received at the hands of callous keepers. His journey through life had been indeed along a *via dolorosa*, the road had been uphill all the way, and now, when the night was at its blackest and the way most steep, he had suddenly found himself, as it were, in a friendly inn, bright with light and warm with welcome. His gratitude to those about him was pathetic in its sincerity and eloquent in the childlike simplicity with which it was expressed.

As I learnt more of this primitive creature I found that there were two anxieties which were prominent in his mind and which he revealed to me with diffidence. He was in the occupation of the rooms assigned to him and had been assured that he would be cared for to the end of his days. This, however, he found hard to realize, for he often asked me timidly to what place he would next be moved. To understand his attitude it is necessary to remember that he had been moving on and moving on all his life. He knew no other state of existence. To him it was normal. He had passed from the workhouse to the hospital, from the hospital back to the workhouse, then from this town to that town or from one show-man's caravan to another. He had never known a home nor any semblance of one. He had no possessions. His sole belongings, besides his clothes and some books, were the monstrous cap and the cloak. He was a wanderer, a pariah and an outcast. That his quarters at the hospital were his for life he could not understand. He could not rid his mind of the anxiety which had pursued him for so many years – where am I to be taken next?

Another trouble was his dread of his fellow-men, his fear of people's eyes, the dread of being always stared at, the lash of the cruel mutterings of the crowd. In his home in Bedstead Square he was secluded; but now and then a thoughtless porter or a wardmaid would open his door to let curious friends have a peep at the Elephant Man. It therefore seemed to him as if the gaze of the world followed him still.

Influenced by these two obsessions he became, during his first few weeks at the hospital, curiously uneasy. At last, with much hesitation, he said to me one day: 'When I am next moved can I go to a blind asylum or to a lighthouse?' He had read about blind asylums in the newspapers and was attracted by the thought of being among people who could not see. The lighthouse had another charm. It meant seclusion from the curious. There at least no one could open a door and peep in at him. Then he would forget that he had once been the Elephant Man. There he would escape the vampire showman. He had never seen a lighthouse, but he had come upon a picture of the Eddystone, and it appeared to him that this lonely column of stone in the waste of the sea was such a home as he had longed for.

I had no great difficulty in ridding Merrick's mind of these ideas. I wanted him to get accustomed to his fellow-men, to become a human being himself and to be admitted to the communion of his kind. He appeared day by day less frightened, less haunted looking, less anxious to hide, less alarmed when he saw his door being opened. He got to know most of the people about the place, to be accustomed to their comings and goings, and to realize that they took no more than a friendly notice of him. He could only go out after dark, and on fine nights ventured to take a walk in Bedstead Square clad in his black cloak and his cap. His greatest adventure was on one moonless evening when he walked alone as far as the hospital garden and back again.

To secure Merrick's recovery and to bring him, as it were, to life once more, it was necessary that he should make the acquaintance of men and women who would treat him as a normal and intelligent young man and not as a monster of deformity. Women I felt to be more important than men in bringing about his transformation. Women were the more frightened of him, the more disgusted at his appearance and the more apt to give way to irrepressible expressions of aversion when they came into his presence. Moreover, Merrick had an admiration of women of such a kind that it attained almost to adoration. This was not the outcome of his personal experience. They were not real women but the products of his imagination. Among them was the beautiful mother surrounded, at a respectful distance, by heroines from the many romances he had read.

His first entry to the hospital was attended by a regrettable incident. He had been placed on the bed in the little attic, and a nurse had been instructed to bring him some food. Unfortunately she had not been fully informed of Merrick's unusual appearance. As she entered the room she saw on the bed, propped up by white pillows, a monstrous figure as hideous as an Indian idol. She at once dropped the tray she was carrying and fled, with a shriek, through the door. Merrick was too weak to notice much, but the experience, I am afraid, was not new to him.

He was looked after by volunteer nurses whose ministrations

were somewhat formal and constrained. Merrick, no doubt, was conscious that their service was purely official, that they were merely doing what they were told to do and that they were acting rather as automata than as women. They did not help him to feel that he was of their kind. On the contrary they, without knowing it, made him aware that the gulf of separation was immeasurable.

Feeling this, I asked a friend of mine, a young and pretty widow, if she thought she could enter Merrick's room with a smile, wish him good morning and shake him by the hand. She said she could and she did. The effect upon poor Merrick was not quite what I had expected. As he let go her hand he bent his head on his knees and sobbed until I thought he would never cease. The interview was over. He told me afterwards that this was the first woman who had ever smiled at him, and the first woman, in the whole of his life, who had shaken hands with him. From this day the transformation of Merrick commenced and he began to change, little by little, from a hunted thing into a man. It was a wonderful change to witness and one that never ceased to fascinate me.

Merrick's case attracted much attention in the papers, with the result that he had a constant succession of visitors. Everybody wanted to see him. He must have been visited by almost every lady of note in the social world. They were all good enough to welcome him with a smile and to shake hands with him. The Merrick whom I had found shivering behind a rag of a curtain in an empty shop was now conversant with duchesses and countesses and other ladies of high degree. They brought him presents, made his room bright with ornaments and pictures, and, what pleased him more than all, supplied him with books. He soon had a large library and most of his day was spent in reading. He was not the least spoiled; not the least puffed up; he never asked for anything; never presumed upon the kindness meted out to him, and was always humbly and profoundly grateful. Above all he lost his shyness. He liked to see his door pushed upon and people look in. He became acquainted with most of the frequenters of Bedstead Square, would chat with them at his window and show them some of his choicest presents. He improved in his speech, although to the end his utterances were not easy for strangers to understand. He was beginning, moreover, to be less conscious of his unsightliness, a little disposed to think it was, after all, not so very extreme. Possibly this was aided by the circumstance that I would not allow a mirror of any kind in his room.

The height of his social development was reached on an eventful day when Queen Alexandra – then Princess of Wales – came to the hospital to pay him a special visit. With that kindness which marked every act of her life, the Queen entered Merrick's room smiling and shook him warmly by the hand. Merrick was transported with delight. This was beyond even his most extravagant dream. The Queen made many people happy, but I think no gracious act of hers ever caused such happiness as she brought into Merrick's room when she sat by his chair and talked to him as to a person she was glad to see.

Merrick, I may say, was now one of the most contented creatures I have chanced to meet. More than once he said to me: 'I am happy every hour of the day.' This was good to think upon when I recalled the half-dead heap of miserable humanity I had seen in the corner of the waiting-room at Liverpool Street. Most men of Merrick's age would have expressed their joy and sense of content-ment by singing or whistling when they were alone. Unfortunately poor Merrick's mouth was so deformed that he could neither whistle nor sing. He was satisfied to express himself by beating time upon the pillow to some tune that was ringing in his head. I have many times found him so occupied when I have entered his room unexpectedly. One thing that always struck me as sad about Merrick was the fact that he could not smile. Whatever his delight might be, his face remained expressionless. He could weep but he could not smile.

The Queen paid Merrick many visits and sent him every year a Christmas card with a message in her own handwriting. On one occasion she sent him a signed photograph of herself. Merrick, quite overcome, regarded it as a sacred object and would hardly allow me to touch it. He cried over it, and after it was framed had it put up in his room as a kind of ikon. I told him that he must write to Her Royal Highness to thank her for her goodness. This he was pleased to do, as he was very fond of writing letters, never before in his life having had anyone to write to. I allowed the letter to be dispatched unedited. It began 'My dear Princess' and ended 'Yours very sincerely'.

Unorthodox as it was it was expressed in terms any courtier would have envied.

Other ladies followed the Queen's gracious example and sent their photographs to this delighted creature who had been all his life despised and rejected of men. His mantelpiece and table became so covered with photographs of handsome ladies, with dainty knicknacks and pretty trifles that they may almost have befitted the apartment of an Adonis-like actor or of a famous tenor.

Through all these bewildering incidents and through the glamour of this great change Merrick still remained in many ways a mere child. He had all the invention of an imaginative boy or girl, the same love of 'make-believe', the same instinct of 'dressing up' and of personating heroic and impressive characters. This attitude of mind was illustrated by the following incident. Benevolent visitors had given me, from time to time, sums of money to be expended for the comfort of the *ci-devant* Elephant Man. When one Christmas was approaching I asked Merrick what he would like me to purchase as a Christmas present. He rather startled me by saying shyly that he would like a dressing-bag with silver fittings. He had seen a picture of such an article in an advertisement which he had furtively preserved.

The association of a silver-fitted dressing-bag with the poor wretch wrapped up in a dirty blanket in an empty shop was hard to comprehend. I fathomed the mystery in time, for Merrick made little secret of the fancies that haunted his boyish brain. Just as a small girl with a tinsel coronet and a window curtain for a train will realize the conception of a countess on her way to court, so Merrick loved to imagine himself a dandy and a young man about town. Mentally, no doubt, he had frequently 'dressed up' for the part. He could 'make-believe' with great effect, but he wanted something to render his fancied character more realistic. Hence the jaunty bag which was to assume the function of the toy coronet and the window curtain that could transform a mite with a pigtail into a countess.

As a theatrical 'property' the dressing-bag was ingenious, since there was little else to give substance to the transformation. Merrick could not wear the silk hat of the dandy nor, indeed, any kind of hat. He could not adapt his body to the trimly cut coat. His deformity was such that he could wear neither collar nor tie, while in association with his bulbous feet the young blood's patent leather shoe was unthinkable. What was there left to make up the character? A lady had given him a ring to wear on his undeformed hand, and a noble lord had presented him with a very stylish walking-stick. But these things, helpful as they were, were hardly sufficing.

The dressing-bag, however, was distinctive, was explanatory and entirely characteristic. So the bag was obtained and Merrick the Elephant Man became in the seclusion of his chamber, the Piccadilly exquisite, the young spark, the gallant, the 'nut'. When I purchased the article I realized that as Merrick could never travel he could hardly want a dressing-bag. He could not use the silver-backed brushes and the comb because he had no hair to brush. The ivory-handled razors were useless because he could not shave. The deformity of his mouth rendered an ordinary toothbrush of no avail, and as his monstrous lips could not hold a cigarette the cigarette-case was a mockery. The silver shoe-horn would be of no service in the putting on of his ungainly slippers, while the hat-brush was quite unsuited to the peaked cap with its visor.

Still the bag was an emblem of the real swell and of the knock-about Don Juan of whom he had read. So every day Merrick laid out upon his table, with proud precision, the silver brushes, the razors, the shoe-horn and the silver cigarette-case which I had taken care to fill with cigarettes. The contemplation of these gave him great pleasure, and such is the power of self-deception that they convinced him he was the 'real thing'.

I think there was just one shadow in Merrick's life. As I have already said, he had a lively imagination; he was romantic; he cherished an emotional regard for women and his favourite pursuit was the reading of love stories. He fell in love – in a humble and devotional way – with, I think, every attractive lady he saw. He, no doubt, pictured himself the hero of many a passionate incident. His bodily deformity had left unmarred the instincts and feelings of his years. He was amorous. He would like to have been a lover, to have walked with the beloved object in the languorous shades of some beautiful garden and to have poured into her ear all the glowing utterances that he had rehearsed in his heart. And yet –

the pity of it! – imagine the feelings of such a youth when he saw nothing but a look of horror creep over the face of every girl whose eyes met his. I fancy when he talked of life among the blind there was a half-formed idea in his mind that he might be able to win the affection of a woman if only she were without eyes to see.

As Merrick developed he began to display certain modest ambitions in the direction of improving his mind and enlarging his knowledge of the world. He was as curious as a child and as eager to learn. There were so many things he wanted to know and see. In the first place he was anxious to view the interior of what he called 'a real house', such a house as figured in many of the tales he knew, a house with a hall, a drawing-room where guests were received and a dining-room with plate on the sideboard and with easy chairs into which the hero could 'fling himself'. The workhouse, the common lodging-house and a variety of mean garrets were all the residences he knew. To satisfy this wish I drove him up to my small house in Wimpole Street. He was absurdly interested and examined everything in detail and with untiring curiosity. I could not show him the pampered menials and the powdered footmen of whom he had read, nor could I produce the white marble staircase of the mansion of romance nor the gilded mirrors and the brocaded divans which belong to that style of residence. I explained that the house was a modest dwelling of the Jane Austen type, and as he had read *Emma* he was content.

A more burning ambition of his was to go to the theatre. It was a project very difficult to satisfy. A popular pantomime was then in progress at Drury Lane Theatre, but the problem was how so conspicuous a being as the Elephant Man could get there, and how he was to see the performance without attracting the notice of the audience and causing a panic or, at least, an unpleasant diversion. The whole matter was most ingeniously carried through by that kindest of women and most able of actresses – Mrs Kendal. She made the necessary arrangements with the lessee of the theatre. A box was obtained. Merrick was brought up in a carriage with drawn blinds and was allowed to make use of the royal entrance so as to reach the box by a private stair. I had begged three of the hospital sisters to don evening dress and to sit in the front row in order to 'dress' the box, on the one hand, and to form a screen for

Merrick on the other. Merrick and I occupied the back of the box which was kept in shadow. All went well, and no one saw a figure, more monstrous than any on the stage, mount the staircase or cross the corridor.

One has often witnessed the unconstrained delight of a child at its first pantomime, but Merrick's rapture was much more intense as well as much more solemn. Here was a being with the brain of a man, the fancies of a youth and the imagination of a child. His attitude was not so much that of delight as of wonder and amazement. He was awed. He was enthralled. The spectacle left him speechless, so that if he were spoken to he took no heed. He often seemed to be panting for breath. I could not help comparing him with a man of his own age in the stalls. This satiated individual was bored to distraction, would look wearily at the stage from time to time and then yawn as if he had not slept for nights; while at the same time Merrick was thrilled by a vision that was almost beyond his comprehension. Merrick talked of this pantomime for weeks and weeks. To him, as to a child with the faculty of make-believe, everything was real; the palace was the home of kings, the princess was of royal blood, the fairies were as undoubted as the children in the street, while the dishes at the banquet were of unquestionable gold. He did not like to discuss it as a play but rather as a vision of some actual world. When this mood possessed him he would say: 'I wonder what the prince did after we left,' or 'Do you think that poor man is still in the dungeon?' and so on and so on.

The splendour and display impressed him, but, I think, the ladies of the ballet took a still greater hold upon his fancy. He did not like the ogres and the giants, while the funny men impressed him as irreverent. Having no experience as a boy of romping and ragging, of practical jokes or of 'larks', he had little sympathy with the doings of the clown, but, I think (moved by some mischievous instinct in his subconscious mind), he was pleased when the policeman was smacked in the face, knocked down and generally rendered undignified.

Later on another longing stirred the depths of Merrick's mind. It was a desire to see the country, a desire to live in some green secluded spot and there learn something about flowers and the ways of animals and birds. The country as viewed from a wagon on a dusty high road was all the country he knew. He had never wandered among the fields nor followed the windings of a wood. He had never climbed to the brow of a breezy down. He had never gathered flowers in a meadow. Since so much of his reading dealt with country life he was possessed by the wish to see the wonders of that life himself.

This involved a difficulty greater than that presented by a visit to the theatre. The project was, however, made possible on this occasion also by the kindness and generosity of a lady – Lady Knightley – who offered Merrick a holiday home in a cottage on her estate. Merrick was conveyed to the railway station in the usual way, but as he could hardly venture to appear on the platform the railway authorities were good enough to run a second-class carriage into a distant siding. To this point Merrick was driven and was placed in the carriage unobserved. The carriage, with the curtains drawn, was then attached to the mainline train.

He duly arrived at the cottage, but the housewife (like the nurse at the hospital) had not been made clearly aware of the unfortunate man's appearance. Thus it happened that when Merrick presented himself his hostess, throwing her apron over her head, fled, gasping, to the fields. She affirmed that such a guest was beyond her powers of endurance for, when she saw him, she was 'that took' as to be in danger of being permanently 'all of a tremble'.

Merrick was then conveyed to a gamekeeper's cottage which was hidden from view and was close to the margin of a wood. The man and his wife were able to tolerate his presence. They treated him with the greatest kindness, and with them he spent the one supreme holiday of his life. He could roam where he pleased. He met no one on his wanderings, for the wood was preserved and denied to all but the gamekeeper and the forester.

There is no doubt that Merrick passed in this retreat the happiest time he had as yet experienced. He was alone in a land of wonders. The breath of the country passed over him like a healing wind. Into the silence of the wood the fearsome voice of the showman could never penetrate. No cruel eyes could peep at him through the friendly undergrowth. It seemed as if in this place of peace all stain had been wiped away from his sullied past. The Merrick who had once crouched terrified in the filthy shadows of a Mile End shop was now sitting in the sun, in a clearing among the trees, arranging a bunch of violets he had gathered.

His letters to me were the letters of a delighted and enthusiastic child. He gave an account of his trivial adventures, of the amazing things he had seen, and of the beautiful sounds he had heard. He had met with strange birds, had startled a hare from her form, had made friends with a fierce dog, and had watched the trout darting in a stream. He sent me some of the wild flowers he had picked. They were of the commonest and most familiar kind, but they were evidently regarded by him as rare and precious specimens.

He came back to London, to his quarters in Bedstead Square, much improved in health, pleased to be 'home' again and to be once more among his books, his treasures and his many friends.

Some six months after Merrick's return from the country he was found dead in bed. This was in April, 1890. He was lying on his back as if asleep, and had evidently died suddenly and without a struggle, since not even the coverlet of the bed was disturbed. The method of his death was peculiar. So large and so heavy was his head that he could not sleep lying down. When he assumed the recumbent position the massive skull was inclined to drop backwards, with the result that he experienced no little distress. The attitude he was compelled to assume when he slept was very strange. He sat up in bed with his back supported by pillows, his knees were drawn up, and his arms clasped round his legs, while his head rested on the points of his bent knees.

He often said to me that he wished he could lie down to sleep 'like other people'. I think on this last night he must, with some determination, have made the experiment. The pillow was soft, and the head, when placed on it, must have fallen backwards and caused a dislocation of the neck. Thus it came about that his death was due to the desire that had dominated his life – the pathetic but hopeless desire to be 'like other people'.

As a specimen of humanity, Merrick was ignoble and repulsive; but the spirit of Merrick, if it could be seen in the form of the living, would assume the figure of an upstanding and heroic man, smooth browed and clean of limb, and with eyes that flashed undaunted courage.

His tortured journey had come to an end. All the way he, like another, had borne on his back a burden almost too grievous to bear. He had been plunged into the Slough of Despond, but with manly steps had gained the farther shore. He had been made 'a spectacle to all men' in the heartless streets of the Vanity Fair. He had been ill-treated and reviled and bespattered with the mud of Disdain. He had escaped the clutches of the Giant Despair, and at last had reached the 'Place of Deliverance', where 'his burden loosed from off his shoulders and fell from off his back, so that he saw it no more.'

Bibliography

1. Books and articles directly relevant to the story of the Elephant Man or his clinical condition

Battiscombe, Georgina, *Queen Alexandra*, Constable, London, 1969.

Bland-Sutton, Sir John, *The Story of a Surgeon*, Methuen, London, 1930.

Boyd, William, *Textbook of Pathology*, Henry Kimpton, London, 1947.

Brain, Russell, *Diseases of the Nervous System*, 5th edition, Oxford University Press, 1956.

Cambridge, 2nd Duke of, *George, Duke of Cambridge: A Memoir of His Private Life, Based on the Journals and Correspondence of H.R.H.*, ed. J. E. Shepherd, 2 vols., Longman, London, 1906.

Carswell, Heather, 'Elephant Man Had More Than Neurofibromatosis', *Journal of the American Medical Association*, vol. 248, no. 9, 3 September 1982, pp. 1032–3; based on *Seminars of Roentgenology*, vol. 17, 1982, p. 153.

Clark, R., 'Proteus Syndrome', in Hughes and Huson (eds.), *Neurofibromatosis*, see below.

Clarke-Kennedy, A. E., *The London: A Study of the Voluntary Hospital System*, vol. 2: *The Second Hundred Years, 1840–1948*, Pitman Medical Publishing, London, 1963.

Cohen Jr, M. Michael, 'Understanding Proteus Syndrome, Unmasking the Elephant Man, and Stemming Elephant Fever', *Neurofibromatosis*, vol. 1, 1988, pp. 260–80.

Crocker, H. Radcliffe, *Diseases of the Skin: a Review of 15,000 Cases of Skin Disorder*, 3rd edition, vol. 2, Lewis, London, 1905.

Crowe, F. W., Schull, W. J., and Neel, J. F., *A Clinical, Pathological and General Study of Multiple Neurofibromatosis*, Charles C. Thomas, Springfield, Ill., 1956.

'Death of the Elephant Man', report in the *British Medical Journal*, vol. I, 16 April 1890, pp. 916–17.

'Death of the Elephant Man', report on inquest in *The Times*, 16 April 1890.

Eaton, Colin, 'Freak Found Refuge on Northants Farm', *Northants Post*, 15 November 1980.

'"Elephant Man", The', report in the *British Medical Journal*, vol. II, 11 December 1886, pp. 1188–9.

Elephant Man, The, pamphlet amplified from an account published in the *British Medical Journal*, John Bale & Sons, London, 1888.

'Elephant Man, The', anonymous article in the *Illustrated Leicester Chronicle,* 27 December 1930.

Entract, J. P., 'The Elephant Man's Pied à Terre', *London Hospital Gazette*, vol. LXXIII, no. 2, May 1970.

Fienman, Norman L., and Yakovac, William C., 'Neurofibromatosis in Childhood', *Journal of Pediatrics*, vol. 76, no. 3, March 1970, pp. 339–46.

Flower, Sir Newman, *Just As It Happened*, Cassell, London, 1950.

Gomm, F. C. Carr, 'Death of the Elephant Man', letter to *The Times*, 16 April 1890.

Gomm, F. C. Carr, 'The Elephant Man', letter of appeal in *The Times*, 4 December 1886.

Graham, Peter W., and Oehlschlaeger, Fritz H., *Articulating the Elephant Man: Joseph Merrick and His Interpreters*, The Johns Hopkins University Press, Baltimore and London, 1992.

Grenfell, Sir Wilfred, *A Labrador Doctor*, revised popular edition, Hodder & Stoughton, London, 1929.

Halsted, D. G., *A Doctor in the Nineties*, Johnson, London, 1959.

Hughes, R. A. C., and Huson, S. (eds.), *Neurofibromatosis*, Chapman & Hall, London (in preparation).

Kaleta, Kenneth C., 'Lynch and History: The Elephant Man', Chapter 2, *David Lynch*, Twayne Publishers, New York, 1992.

Kendal, Madge, *Dame Madge Kendal by Herself*, John Murray, London, 1933.

Merrick, Joseph Carey, *The Autobiography of Joseph Carey Merrick*, H. & A. Cockshaw, Leicester, n.d.

Minutes of the London Hospital House Committee, 7 December 1886; 14 December 1886; 15 April 1890.

Montagu, Ashley, *The Elephant Man: A Study in Human Dignity*, Allison & Busby, London, 1972; Outerbridge & Dienstfrey, New York, 1971.

Norman, Tom, 'This is Tom Norman: Sixty-five Years a Showman and Auctioneer', unpublished MS in possession of the Norman family; subsequently published as *The Penny Showman: Memoirs of Tom Norman, 'Silver King'*, with additional writings by his son, George Barnum Norman, privately printed, London, 1985.

Norman, Tom, letter of self-justification in the *World's Fair*, 24 February 1923.

Poole, E. F., *The Story of Byfield*, Archer & Goodman, Northampton, 1930; this repeats an article, 'The Romance of Redhill Wood', *Northampton County Magazine*, vol. I, 1928, pp. 292–3.

Reed, Nicholas, 'The Mystery of Lot 583', *World Medicine*, 29 November 1980.

Reports of the first meeting of the Pathological Society of London to consider the case of the Elephant Man, *British Medical Journal*, vol. II, 6 December 1884, p. 1140; *Lancet*, vol. II, 6 December 1884, p. 1000; of the second meeting, *British Medical Journal*, vol. I, 21 March 1885, p. 595; *Lancet*, vol. I, 21 March 1885, pp. 1188–9.

Reviews of *The Elephant Man and Other Reminiscences* by Sir Frederick Treves, *British Medical Journal*, vol. I, 17 March 1923, p. 335; *Lancet*, vol. I, 17 March 1923, pp. 547–8; *World's Fair*, 10 February 1923.

Seward, G. R., 'The Elephant Man', Parts I-III, *British Dental Journal*, 22 September 1990, pp. 173–5; 6 October 1990, pp. 209–16; 20 October 1990, pp. 252–5.

Seward, G. R., 'Joseph Merrick', in Hughes and Huson (eds.), op. cit.

Somerset, Lady Geraldine, 'Private Journal of the Duchess of Cambridge', MS diary in the Royal Archives, Windsor Castle Library.

Tibbles, J. A. R., and Cohen Jr, M. M., 'The Proteus Syndrome: the Elephant Man Diagnosed', *British Medical Journal*, vol. 293, 13 September 1986.

Treves, Frederick, 'A Case of Congenital Deformity', *Transactions of the Pathological Society of London*, vol. XXXVI, 1885, pp. 494–8.

Treves, Sir Frederick, *The Elephant Man and Other Reminiscences*, Cassell, London, 1923.

Trombley, Stephen, *Sir Frederick Treves: The Extra-Ordinary Edwardian*, Routledge, London, 1989.

Weber, F. Parkes, 'Cutaneous Pigmentation as an Incomplete Form of Recklinghausen's Disease, with Remarks on the Classification of Incomplete Forms of Recklinghausen's Disease', *British Journal of Dermatology*, vol. 21, 1949, pp. 49–51.

Weber, F. Parkes, *Further Rare Diseases and Debatable Subjects*, Staples Press, London, 1949.

Weber, F. Parkes, 'Periosteal Neurofibromatosis, with a Short Consideration of the Whole Subject of Neurofibromatosis', *Quarterly Journal of Medicine*, vol. 23, 1930, p. 151.

Wiedemann, H.-R., Burgio, G. R., Aldenhoff, P., Kunze, J., Kaufmann, H. J., and Schirg, E., 'The Proteus Syndrome', *European Journal of Pediatrics*, vol. 140, 1983, pp. 5–12.

Wilson, S. A. Kinnier, *Neurology*, vol. 2, Arnold, London, 1940.

The story of Joseph Merrick in Treves's version provided the inspiration for the play by Bernard Pomerance, *The Elephant Man*, first produced at the Hampstead Theatre, London, in 1977, and later on Broadway and at the National Theatre in London; text published by Faber & Faber, London, 1980. Treves's story was, as well, the starting point for the script of the film also called *The Elephant Man* (directed by David Lynch, starring John Hurt) which was released in 1980.

2. Selected list of other works consulted

'A Palace of Varieties for Leicester', *Nottingham Journal*, 3 September 1883.

Altick, Richard, *The Shows of London*, Belknap Press of Harvard University Press, 1978.

Cullen, Tom, *The Times and Crimes of Jack the Ripper* (originally entitled *Autumn of Terror*), Fontana, London, 1966.

Dallas, Duncan, *The Travelling People*, Macmillan, London, 1971.

Ellis, Colin D. B., *History in Leicester*, 2nd edition, City of Leicester Information Department, 1969.

Ellis, I. C., *Nineteenth Century Leicester*, Leicester, n.d.

Evans, Bergen, *The Natural History of Nonsense*, Michael Joseph, London, 1947.

Frost, Thomas, *The Old Showmen and the Old London Fairs*, Tinsley Brothers, London, 1874.

Hardwicke, Sir Cedric, *A Victorian in Orbit*, Methuen, London, 1961.

Hardy, Florence Emily, *The Life of Thomas Hardy, 1840–1928*, Macmillan, London, 1962.

Hone, William, 'The Editor's Visits to Claude Amboise Seurat', 26 July 1825; 'Visit to Bartholomew Fair', 5 September 1825; *The Every-day Book*, new edition, vol. I, Thomas Tegg, London, 1841.

'Mr Sam Torr', *Music Hall*, 23 February 1889.

Morley, Henry, *Memoirs of Bartholomew Fair*, new edition, Chatto & Windus, London, 1880.

Obituary notices of Sir Frederick Treves: *British Medical Journal*, vol. II, 15 December 1923, pp. 1185–9; *Lancet*, vol. II, 15 December 1923, p. 1325; *The Times*, 10 December 1923.

Porter, Enid, *Cambridgeshire Customs and Folklore*, Routledge & Kegan Paul, London, 1969.

Porter, Enid, *The Folklore of East Anglia*, Batsford, London, 1974.

Reviews of the pantomime, *The Babes in the Wood*: *Illustrated London News*, 7 January 1888; *Punch*, 7 January 1888.

'Tom Norman', *The Era*, 26 October 1901.

Torr, Clara, MS diary in possession of the Torr family.

Treves, Sir Frederick, *Highways and Byways in Dorset*, Macmillan, London, 1906.

Treves, Sir Frederick, *The Other Side of the Lantern*, Cassell, London, 1905.

Tyrwhitt-Drake, Sir Garrard, *The English Circus and Fairground*, Methuen, London, 1946.

Viski, Károly, *Hungarian Peasant Customs*, 2nd edition, George Vajnu, Budapest, 1937.

Wilson, A. E., *Christmas Pantomime*, Allen & Unwin, London, 1934.

Index

Discover more about our forthcoming books through Penguin's FREE newspaper...

Penguin
Quarterly

It's packed with:

- exciting features
- author interviews
- previews & reviews
- books from your favourite films & TV series
- exclusive competitions & much, much more...

FOR THE BEST IN PAPERBACKS, LOOK FOR THE 🐧

In every corner of the world, on every subject under the sun, Penguin represents quality and variety – the very best in publishing today.

For complete information about books available from Penguin – including Puffins, Penguin Classics and Arkana – and how to order them, write to us at the appropriate address below. Please note that for copyright reasons the selection of books varies from country to country.

In the United Kingdom: Please write to *Dept JC, Penguin Books Ltd, FREEPOST, West Drayton, Middlesex, UB7 0BR.*

If you have any difficulty in obtaining a title, please send your order with the correct money, plus ten per cent for postage and packaging, to *PO Box No 11, West Drayton, Middlesex*

In the United States: Please write to *Dept BA, Penguin, 299 Murray Hill Parkway, East Rutherford, New Jersey 07073*

In Canada: Please write to *Penguin Books Canada Ltd, 2801 John Street, Markham, Ontario L3R 1B4*

In Australia: Please write to the *Marketing Department, Penguin Books Australia Ltd, P.O. Box 257, Ringwood, Victoria 3134*

In New Zealand: Please write to the *Marketing Department, Penguin Books (NZ) Ltd, Private Bag, Takapuna, Auckland 9*

In India: Please write to *Penguin Overseas Ltd, 706 Eros Apartments, 56 Nehru Place, New Delhi, 110019*

In the Netherlands: Please write to *Penguin Books Netherlands B.V., Postbus 3507, NL–1001 AH, Amsterdam*

In West Germany: Please write to *Penguin Books Ltd, Friedrichstrasse 10–12, D–6000 Frankfurt/Main 1*

In Spain: Please write to *Alhambra Longman S.A., Fernandez de la Hoz 9, E–28010 Madrid*

In Italy: Please write to *Penguin Italia s.r.l., Via Como 4, I-20096 Pioltello (Milano)*

In France: Please write to *Penguin France S.A., 17 rue Lejeune, F-31000 Toulouse*

In Japan: Please write to *Longman Penguin Japan Co Ltd, Yamaguchi Building, 2–12–9 Kanda Jimbocho, Chiyoda-Ku, Tokyo 101*

FOR THE BEST IN PAPERBACKS, LOOK FOR THE 🐧

A CHOICE OF PENGUINS

Riding the Iron Rooster Paul Theroux

An eye-opening and entertaining account of travels in old and new China, from the author of *The Great Railway Bazaar*. 'Mr Theroux cannot write badly ... in the course of a year there was almost no train in the vast Chinese rail network on which he did not travel' – Ludovic Kennedy

The Life of Graham Greene Norman Sherry
Volume One 1904–1939

'Probably the best biography ever of a living author' – Philip French in the *Listener*. Graham Greene has always maintained a discreet distance from his reading public. This volume reconstructs his first thirty-five years to create one of the most revealing literary biographies of the decade.

The Chinese David Bonavia

'I can think of no other work which so urbanely and entertainingly succeeds in introducing the general Western reader to China' – *Sunday Telegraph*

All the Wrong Places James Fenton

Who else but James Fenton could have played a Bach prelude on the presidential piano – and stolen one of Imelda's towels – on the very day Marcos left his palace in Manila? 'He is the most professional of amateur war correspondents, a true though unusual journo, top of the trade. When he arrives in town, prudent dictators pack their bags and quit' – *The Times*

Voices of the Old Sea Norman Lewis

'Limpidly and lovingly, Norman Lewis has caught the helpless, unwitting, often foolish, but always hopeful village in its dying summers, and saved the tragedy with sublime comedy' – *Observer*

Ninety-Two Days Evelyn Waugh

With characteristic honesty, Evelyn Waugh here debunks the romantic notions attached to rough travelling. His journey in Guiana and Brazil is difficult, dangerous and extremely uncomfortable, and his account of it is witty and unquestionably compelling.

A CHOICE OF PENGUINS

The Assassination of Federico García Lorca   Ian Gibson

Lorca's 'crime' was his antipathy to pomposity, conformity and intolerance. His punishment was murder. Ian Gibson – author of the acclaimed new biography of Lorca – reveals the truth about his death and the atmosphere in Spain that allowed it to happen.

Between the Woods and the Water   Patrick Leigh Fermor

Patrick Leigh Fermor continues his celebrated account – begun in *A Time of Gifts* – of his journey on foot from the Hook of Holland to Constantinople. 'Even better than everyone says it is' – Peter Levi. 'Indescribably rich and beautiful' – *Guardian*

The Time Out Film Guide   Edited by Tom Milne

The definitive, up-to-the-minute directory of 9,000 films – world cinema from classics and silent epics to reissues and the latest releases – assessed by two decades of *Time Out* reviewers. 'In my opinion the best and most comprehensive' – Barry Norman

Metamagical Themas   Douglas R. Hofstadter

This astonishing sequel to the bestselling, Pulitzer Prize-winning *Gödel, Escher, Bach* swarms with 'extraordinary ideas, brilliant fables, deep philosophical questions and Carrollian word play' – Martin Gardner

Into the Heart of Borneo   Redmond O'Hanlon

'Perceptive, hilarious and at the same time a serious natural-history journey into one of the last remaining unspoilt paradises' – *New Statesman*. 'Consistently exciting, often funny and erudite without ever being overwhelming' – *Punch*

When the Wind Blows   Raymond Briggs

'A visual parable against nuclear war: all the more chilling for being in the form of a strip cartoon' – *Sunday Times*. 'The most eloquent anti-Bomb statement you are likely to read' – *Daily Mail*

FOR THE BEST IN PAPERBACKS, LOOK FOR THE 🐧

A CHOICE OF PENGUINS

Brian Epstein: The Man Who Made the Beatles   Ray Coleman

'An excellent biography of Brian Epstein, the lonely, gifted man whose artistic faith and bond with the Beatles never wavered – and whose recognition of genius created a cultural era, even though it destroyed him' – *Mail on Sunday*

A Thief in the Night   John Cornwell

A veil of suspicion and secrecy surrounds the last hours of Pope John Paul I, whose thirty-three day reign ended in a reported heart attack on the night of 28 September 1978. Award-winning crime writer John Cornwell was invited by the Vatican to investigate. 'The best detective story you will ever read' – *Daily Mail*

Among the Russians   Colin Thubron

One man's solitary journey by car across Russia provides an enthralling and revealing account of the habits and idiosyncrasies of a fascinating people. 'He sees things with the freshness of an innocent and the erudition of a scholar' – *Daily Telegraph*

Higher than Hope   Fatima Meer

The authorized biography of Nelson Mandela. 'An astonishing read ... the most complete, authoritative and moving tribute thus far' – *Time Out*

Stones of Aran: Pilgrimage   Tim Robinson

Arainn is the largest of the three Aran Islands, and one of the world's oldest landscapes. This 'wholly irresistible' (*Observer*) and uncategorizable book charts a sunwise journey around its coast – and explores an open secret, teasing out the paradoxes of a terrain at once bare and densely inscribed.

Bernard Shaw   Michael Holroyd
Volume I 1856–1898: The Search for Love

'In every sense, a spectacular piece of work ... A feat of style as much as of research, which will surely make it a flamboyant new landmark in modern English life-writing' – Richard Holmes in *The Times*